beginner's guide to
yoga

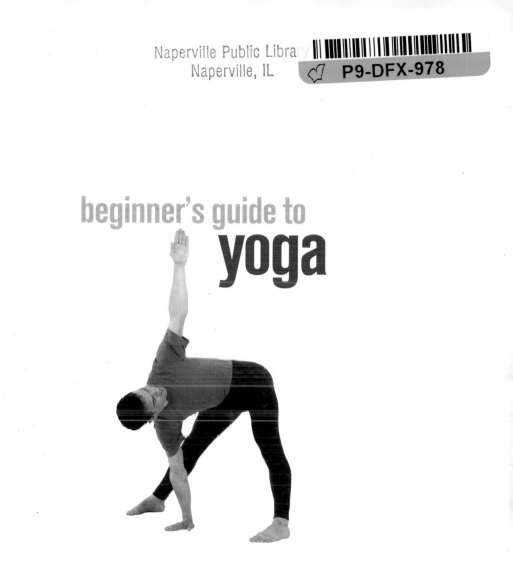

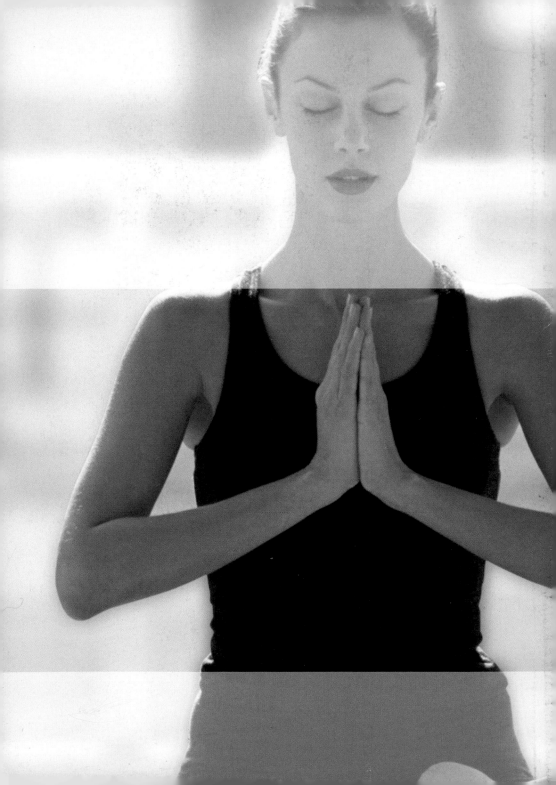

beginner's guide to
yoga

HOWARD KENT & CLAIRE HAYLER

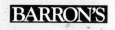

First edition for the United States,
its territories and dependencies, and
Canada published in 2003
by Barron's Educational Series, Inc.

Conceived and created by
Axis Publishing Limited
8c Accommodation Road
London NW11 8ED
www.axispublishing.co.uk

Creative Director: Siân Keogh
Design: Axis Design Editions
Managing Editor: Conor Kilgallon
Editorial Director: Brian Burns
Production Manager: Tim Clarke
Photographer: Mike Good

NOTE
The opinions and advice expressed in
this book are intended as a guide only.
The publisher and author accept no
responsibility for any injury or loss
sustained as a result of using this book.

All inquiries should be addressed to:
Barron's Educational Series, Inc.
250 Wireless Boulevard
Hauppauge, New York 11788
http://www.barronseduc.com

Library of Congress Catalog Card No:
2002116913

ISBN 0–7641–2582–6

9 8 7 6 5 4 3 2 1

Printed and bound in Singapore

contents

beginner's guide to **yoga**

introduction

Ever since man began to communicate through language, developing the capacity to think objectively, the puzzle of existence has played on the human mind, which has constantly sought explanations for both life and death. Central to any explanation are the questions, "Who am I?" and "What is my role in life?"

Regular practice of yoga enriches the inner life, releasing the mind from everyday stress and the restrictions of the body, and bringing peace and personal fulfillment.

what yoga means

The birth and growth of what we now know as yoga first started around 5,000 years ago in northern India and although many parts of its history are unclear, we are able to piece together certain remarkable facts. The word yoga comes from the classical Sanskrit language used in ancient India and is generally translated as "union."

However, the practice of yoga developed many centuries after the word itself came into use. What it actually means is "to yoke" and it is an assertion that although we live in a world of millions of apparently separate phenomena—matter, people, animals, plants, thoughts, and ideas—in fact, everything is a part of a single, great whole.

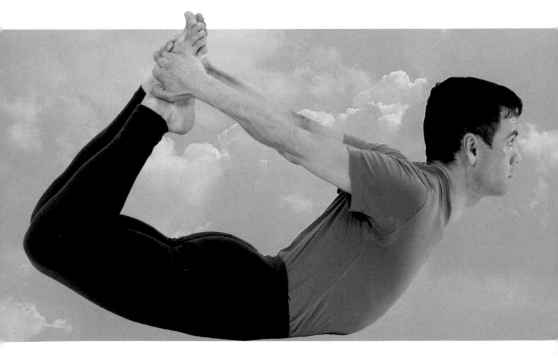

understanding through stillness

In their search, the yogis discovered the importance of stillness, both physical and mental. A great sage of yoga, Patanjali, declared some 2,000 years ago: "Yoga is controlling the waves of the mind." This, however, we know to be extremely difficult—our minds are more often like chattering monkeys.

So the yogis first examined stillness in the body. Being used to sitting on the ground, they experimented with different ways of doing this and came up with what they called the asana (pronounced "ah-sna"), which translates as "holding a position." This manifests itself in several ways, from the universally known headstand, to simply sitting correctly on a chair. The essentials of the asanas will be discussed later (pp. 36–79).

What the yogis found was that if they sat correctly, slowed the breath, and calmed the mind, they gained great insights into life. Amazingly, they almost all came to the same conclusions. They learned intuitively that the basis of everything we call existence is a force, which came to be known as brahman. This force is not a human force but a universal force of consciousness, which they called purusha. This cosmic force was interwoven with prakriti, the material substance of the universe. Human beings, they understood, are an integral part of this interweaving—precisely what Einstein was postulating.

WIDENING THE CIRCLE

Consider the words of Albert Einstein, the greatest scientist our civilization has produced, who wrote:
"A human being is a part of the whole called by us 'the universe,' a part limited in time and space. He experiences himself, his thoughts and feelings, as something separate from the rest—a kind of optical delusion of his consciousness... Our task must be to free ourselves from this prison by widening our circle and compassion to embrace all living creatures and the whole of nature in its beauty."
This is exactly the conclusion the early yogis came to, thousands of years ago.

the part and the whole

A sense of isolation from the world and separation from our true selves is at the center of all our suffering. Yoga complements other spiritual teachings that tell us we are all part of an undivided whole. The development of yoga practice helps us to further understand this, not merely intellectually, but also integrally, thus transforming our lives. While there are many different aspects of yoga, known as the eight limbs (see pp. 18–19), they all form part of a whole. Thus the asanas are not merely physical exercises, but work on every aspect of our life. This makes yoga unique.

the enduring value of yoga

Exercise programs and philosophical concepts come and go, but yoga persists and its practice is now growing at an unparalleled rate. It is remarkable how many people have studied the subject seriously, transforming their own lives and the lives of others.

what can yoga offer me?

The first thing yoga can offer is a sense of calmness and peace of mind. These are the things we need most in life. We can be fit and physically healthy, but still unhappy, worried, and strained. Everything about yoga aims at developing serenity.

stress relief

In recent years, more and more has been learned about the degree to which the body is controlled by the mind. One of the most frequently used words in our society is "stress." Life, we complain, is so stressful.

It is strange to consider then that the word "stress" did not exist in relation to human activity until it was first used 60 years ago by the Austrian-born scientist Professor Hans Selye.

At the same time that stress research has developed, scientists have also looked into how the immune system works. Experiments in this area show that the immune system works best in a relaxed, peaceful individual, rather than in a stressed, angry, or frightened one. So a sense of peace in life is actually beneficial to human beings' physical health.

the mind–body connection

The interplay between body and mind is still undervalued. To illustrate this, two psychologists in Manchester, England, brought together a group of people for an experiment. All members of the group had to press one finger firmly against a tabletop. The group was then divided into three: one section was told to forget the whole experiment, the second had to carry out the same physical action once a week, and the third was told not to carry it out but simply to recall the experience mentally once a week.

After eight weeks the group was retested. The first section showed no change, the second had improved muscle tone by about a third, but, most interestingly, the third group showed an improvement of about 15 percent, without having used their muscles physically at all. So their mental activity was capable of producing a significant physical result.

The American surgeon, Bernie Siegel, who has written of the power of the heart and mind in fighting cancer, has said: "Every thought you have goes into every cell in your body." Compare that with the statement of Patanjali, already quoted, that yoga involves controlling the waves of the mind, and you can see how current research demonstrates the fundamental truth of yoga.

Many people complain that controlling the mind is very difficult. Consider, however, the implications of this: if we cannot control the mind, it means that we are out of control. If we are out of control, then it becomes easy to see how life can overwhelm us.

In the United States, the Occupational Stress Research Institute estimates that stress costs industry some $150 billion a year. In Britain, it is estimated that £8 billion ($12 billion) is lost annually as a result of work time lost through stress factors.

A POWER TO USE WISELY

There is—or should be—no fanaticism in yoga. In India there are holy men called *fakirs*. Some of them have shown their devotion to God by curling their fingers, raising their arm, and keeping it raised—for the rest of their lives. The pain will initially be excruciating, but eventually the arm will stiffen and be immovable. Although this seems extreme, it does show how mind and body can be controlled and linked. The path of moderation is the best one to follow with any yoga practice and the mind–body link that yoga provides can make life happier and healthier, not just for ourselves but for all. Again, let us emphasize that this is not make-believe; it is a matter of actual experience and research.

a different kind of exercise

To understand the benefits of yoga, we need to keep the word "unity" in mind: unity in life itself—the word the Buddhists use is "compassion"—and unity in all our actions.

Let us take the example of the asana, or posture. Most exercise programs focus wholly on the physical movement or pose and largely ignore the mind; you can exercise your body while thinking about what you are going to cook for supper. At this level, the yoga asana is beneficial, but not remarkable, and it is clear that there is no link between mind and body, which will inevitably result in confusion between the two.

However, properly executed, the asana brings together the physical movement with the coordination of the breathing, concentration on the parts of the body being used, and a harmonious state of mind linking all these aspects. The difference in the result is enormous.

mind and motion
When you come to study the program of asanas later in the book, you will find that many are static, others involve slow, controlled movement, and just a few involve a sudden, strong movement. By joining mind with motion, beneficial changes occur, not merely physically but also mentally, in the form of relaxation. This link has proved useful when dealing with ill health and yoga is also used to help those with a range of life-threatening illnesses such as cancer, multiple sclerosis (MS), or Parkinson's disease. Despite the severity of these conditions, a balanced program of asanas, enhanced breathing, and increased mental stability has often been found to lead to considerable improvements taking place.

YOGA FOR ALL

Yoga can help you achieve more than you think possible, regardless of issues such as weight, age, disability, or physical condition:

- Many older people find yoga helps maintain or even restore mobility to the body. It may also help prevent many illnesses associated with old age.

- People with disabilities can benefit just as much from yoga as those who are able-bodied.

- Pregnant women find gentle stretching and breathing help relieve some of the physical discomforts associated with pregnancy and help prepare them for labor. Special yoga classes are also available for pregnant women.

- Children over five years of age can benefit from learning to breathe and relax—valuable in later life.

The secret is never to push yourself unduly. If your body tells you to stop, do so immediately.

self-appreciation

Usually, the first objective in taking up yoga is personal benefit. If your practice is based on an appreciation of yoga as union, it will soon become apparent that the best way to find yourself is actually to lose yourself first. To add to the apparent contradiction, it must also be seen that we can lose ourselves only if we appreciate ourselves, in other words, to understand that we are an essential part of the union. It is important to stress that yoga is unconditional union, not because we think everybody and everything should be agreeable to us, but because everything is inextricably a part of the whole.

It is useful to liken human life to the running of a well-managed company. To be effective, the head of the company needs to have experience far beyond the specific requirements of his or her particular job. Our realization that we are part of a whole is that experience.

The first objective of yoga, therefore, is to love ourselves—but not in a self-absorbed, narcissistic way. The more we learn of the whole, the more we understand the individuals making up that whole. The more we isolate ourselves from others, the more unhappy and irritable we become.

a journey, not a race

The aspect of yoga involving static and dynamic poses is a style called "Hatha yoga." The slow, relaxed pace is central to its success. Periods of mental and physical relaxation keep the central purpose before us.

APPRECIATING OUR BODIES

Our bodies contain countless cells and they are all programmed to do a specific job. Constant nagging or complaining will lead to inefficiency. The right sort of encouragement will stimulate those cells. For example, when something goes wrong physically, we tend to complain. If a knee hurts, we are tempted to castigate it for being injured. From our knowledge of the workings of the human body's repair systems, however, we know that the knee tries to develop and keep itself fit at all times. A variety of things may have combined to interfere with its efficient working—genetics, the conditions under which it is made to work, and so on—but the knee itself continues to work to maintain its fitness. Our complaining about it only makes its task harder.

the benefits of yoga

In addition to remembering the wholeness aspect of yoga, regular practice can improve many specific mental and physical issues. Yoga:

■ Realigns the entire body, encouraging good posture. It strengthens the bones and muscles and increases mobility in the joints.

■ Encourages flexibility and reduces back pain through frequent stretching and exercising. This is especially important because human beings experience an immense range of spinal problems, not because of bad body design but because of lifestyle factors.

■ Improves blood circulation and oxygenation through better breathing.

■ Increases vitality and energy levels.

■ Massages internal organs, improving their function. Digestion is improved as better breathing stimulates the abdominal organs.

■ Calms the mind and soothes the emotions, relieving stress and anxiety.

■ Enables clear and focused thinking through increased oxygen supply to the brain. Clear thinking builds self-confidence and self-esteem.

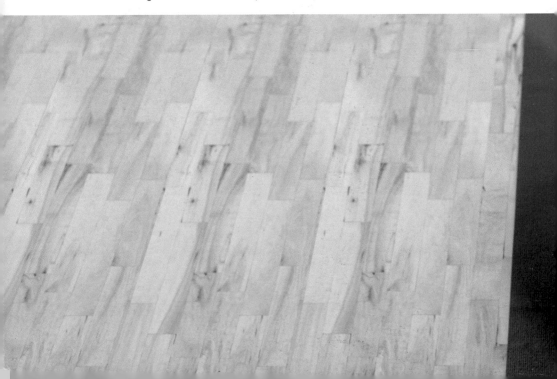

1	Yoga is not about admiring ourselves.
2	Yoga is not about achievement or competing with other students; don't get upset if you can't perform a certain exercise.
3	Yoga does not try to fit us all into one mold; it respects our differences, mentally and physically. Some of the finest yoga teachers have only a very limited ability in practicing the postures. Of these, a number suffer from a chronic disability, yet their study and approach enables them to show more able-bodied people the way forward.
4	Yoga takes patience and quiet persistence, learning not to become discouraged when a fellow classmate can stretch further or hold a pose longer.

So be gentle with yourself and realize you cannot accomplish everything in a day.

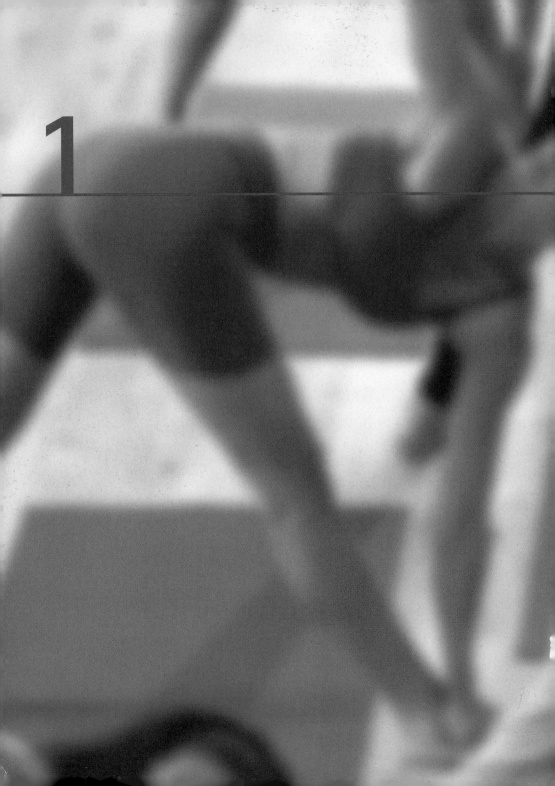

1

fundamental principles

To get the maximum benefit from yoga, it is best to begin by being aware of the principles upon which you should build your practice. These include the eight limbs of Classical yoga, the importance of ethical living, and the realization that yoga is not competitive or goal driven but is, instead, a discipline based on cooperation and reconciliation. On a day-to-day basis, this is supported by regular practice, controlling breathing, undoing ingrained bad habits, and controlling the mind through concentration, contemplation, and deep meditation.

the eight limbs of yoga

With such a wide relevance to all aspects of life, yoga can manifest itself in many ways. This is particularly true in the West, where yoga practice has developed only over the past 30 or 40 years, in, of course, a totally different type of society from that in which it originated. Inevitably, therefore, yoga teachings will, to some degree, be adapted to the times. The fundamental principles of yoga remain constant even if the external applications take different forms.

core ideas

The yoga propounded by Patanjali and other sages is called "Raja yoga"—the King of Yogas. This, as we have already seen, places the emphasis firmly on controlling the mind. It can also be described as Classical yoga. Although there are different ancient schools of yoga (see pp. 92–93), they all share certain common principles. They are not separate entities but involve differences in emphasis.

The early sages appear to have been of one mind on a number of points. Of central importance is that all students start by taking an ethical approach to life. The sages also all agree on the importance of breathing, of the poses, and of meditative and concentration practices, but equally they insist these will all be useless unless we first address ourselves to our ethical standards.

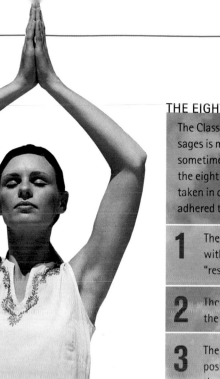

THE EIGHT LIMBS

The Classical yoga of Patanjali and the other early sages is made up of eight parts. That is why it is also sometimes referred to as "Ashtanga yoga"—the yoga of the eight limbs, or steps. To some degree these are to be taken in order but this recommendation need not be adhered to with complete rigidity.

1 The *yamas* (the five observances), which along with the *niyamas* (see below) are often called the "restraints," and are rules of conduct.

2 The *niyamas* (the five actions) complement the yamas.

3 The asanas, which originally applied to a sitting position for the quieting of the mind—the basis of the practice of yoga. They also increase physical well-being through the practice of an integrated set of physical exercises.

4 *Pranayama* is the control of the life force (*prana*) through the breath.

5 *Pratyahara* is the necessity of not being a slave to the senses of the outer world, and leads to examining the essential inner world contained within us all.

6 *Darana* is the development of single-minded concentration, the first step in meditation.

7 *Dyana* is the deeper process of contemplation and meditation, the heart of yoga.

8 *Samadi* is the ultimate state of deep meditation and is bliss, unity, and transcendence. The ego is left behind and the soul is liberated.

yoga and ethical values

The ethical standards of yoga are called *yamas*, the way we interact with others, and *niyamas*, the way we conduct our own lives. We are abjured not to be violent, in thought, word, or deed (*ahimsa* is the name for this principle of nonviolence), not to be covetous, not to steal, to face life with equanimity, to be clean in all ways, and to live a life of love, not lust.

It may seem a tall order to embrace all this in order to practice yoga postures or carry out breathing exercises. The insistence of Classical yoga on ethical considerations does not mean, however, that in order to take up yoga practice we have to become a saint or a philosopher. We do need to realize, though, that if our own outlook is not peaceful and creative, then the various aspects of our life will be at war with each other and no amount of exercising or controlled breathing will do any good. We need to understand the ends to which we are working and to include progress in these areas in our day-by-day approach.

nonviolence

The amount of violence and antagonism in our society today is truly dispiriting, but how are we to cope with it? The word "rage" crops up everywhere. Then rage creates responsive rage, and so on. Buddha declared: "Hate never conquered hate—only love conquers hate." This may sound like wishful thinking, but in fact it demands courage and strength of purpose.

The Classical yoga approach, therefore, is based on the understanding that while competition may have a role in life, the overwhelming necessity is cooperation. If we do not seek to reduce the spirit of competition, then antagonism within our own body and mind will grow and no amount of exercise will eradicate it; on the contrary, it may well be enhanced.

anger management

In the United States, there is an organization known as the SYDA Prison Project that provides a home study course called "In Search of the Self," free of charge to any prisoner who requests it. The lessons explain the timeless wisdom of yoga and meditation. Currently, over 4,000 inmates are enrolled. Swami Muktananda, who founded the project in 1979, wrote to prisoners, saying, "If you want to respect yourself, if you want to improve yourself, if you want to experience the joy of your own inner self, you can do that anywhere, even in prison." Other meditation-based organizations include the Prison Smart Los Angeles Youth Project and the Human Kindness Institute.

Similarly, in Britain, the Prison Phoenix Trust runs classes in yoga and meditation in prisons. The prisoners who participate include many with long sentences, often for violent offenses. Many respond to this approach, which is based on reconciliation rather than revenge.

controlling our breathing

After the ethical standards and the asanas (the physical postures), comes the fourth part of Classical yoga: *pranayama*, controlling our breathing. We must remember that the way we look at life does not merely affect our emotions; it also affects us physically to a degree that we profoundly underestimate. Breath control will be examined in more detail later in this book, but it must be emphasized that as we are, so will we breathe. If we are frightened, our breath will come in gasps. If we are angry, the body tenses and the breath is stifled. If we could see a chart showing how our breathing changes with our emotions, we would be amazed.

Through the practice of yoga, we find that as we breathe, so can we become; by controlling our breathing, we can begin to control our emotions. Regular, effective, free breathing is central to mental and physical peace, and the conglomeration of emotional signals we give out day by day connects intimately with all aspects of our health.

YOGA EVERY DAY

First thing in the morning, it's a good idea to exercise our bodies gently. Not only does yoga loosen up our bodies, but it sharpens our outlook for the day. How we feel mentally on waking will depend on a number of factors: how well we slept, the dreams we had, any unresolved problems that are worrying us, and so on. The important thing to remember is that yoga can help us move through any mental or emotional state that we may face throughout the day.

It takes only a little forethought to see that we should start the day in the right way. On waking, a few gentle stretches, performed thoughtfully, should be accompanied by breathing a little more deeply, slowly, and rhythmically. Then we can remind ourselves that only the moment in which we are living now has any reality.

What we get out of the day will, to quite a degree, depend on how we look at and accept situations as they unfold. So, while the movement and the breathing are helpful, the key lies in the mental state in which they are performed. We attempt to face life with equanimity or dispassion, dealing as evenly as possible with our positive or negative impressions of life.

It is also a good idea to take just a few minutes, from time to time, during the day, to repeat this practice. This is quite apart from any personal or group yoga session that we may be involved in. The effect of repeating this simple practice throughout the day can help us put our "good" and "bad" experiences into perspective.

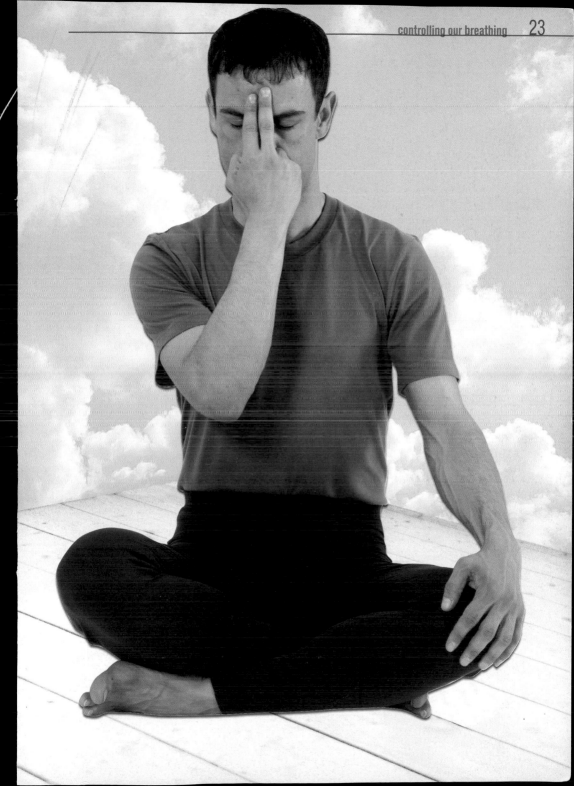

controlling the senses

The need to master our senses and emotions and not to allow ourselves to be their slave, *pratyahara*, is the fifth part of Classical yoga. Controlling the senses is a matter not of suppression but of rising above. Many of our reactions are habits that have developed over the years—and habits are hard to break. If, however, we feel that we can't break them, we are again saying that life controls us, not that we—to a substantial degree—control life. As has already been seen, such an outlook can lead to great difficulties.

blame

One very common habitual reaction to adverse circumstances is to look for something or someone to blame—the traffic, your boss, or the weather. A lovely word in Sanskrit is *santosha*, which means "equanimity"—realizing that we all have a role in the situations in which we find ourselves and that simply trying to lay the blame elsewhere is not only useless but damaging. Looking for other people or factors to blame actually harms us.

It is critical to appreciate the link between our breath and our thoughts. Dispassion does not mean having no opinion or attitude, but ensuring that our responses are constructive rather then destructive.

Controlling the senses also extends to sexual attraction. Most of the world's deepest teachings have

considered the problem caused by sexual attraction, and many adherents of different religions have embraced chastity. Some yoga teachings have been interpreted in this manner but examination shows that what is being said is that sexual activity needs to be a

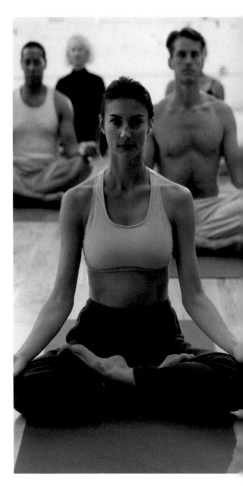

central aspect of the amazing process we call love and not merely an expression of lust. Of course our particular situation will also determine our sexual behavior. What is true for the majority of us may not be true for someone such as an ordained monk.

controlling the mind

The last three steps of Classical yoga—*darana*, *dyana*, and *samadi*—are all mental stages, usually interpreted as concentration, contemplation, and deep meditation.

We all need the ability to concentrate and this plays a central part in all the aspects. Asanas or breathing exercises without concentration are of little value, and if we are gradually going to gain control over our lives and activities, this can be achieved only with a developed ability to be single-minded in both thought and action.

A major difficulty is that we often expect results immediately, but this is unrealistic. The ability to be quietly persistent is therefore invaluable. Only then will we begin to see results. We realize intuitively that something valuable is taking place within us.

Dyana, the meditative state, is attained when the mind concentrates and becomes absorbed in an object of focus. Meditation is at the very heart of yoga. The famous German writer Johann Wolfgang von Goethe neatly summed up the idea: "Be attentive to the present. Only in the present time can we understand eternity."

Finally, yoga can take us to a state of bliss, unity, and transcendence of time and space. This is the ultimate goal of yoga and a culmination of the seven previous limbs. *Samadi* is attained when the ego is conquered and the soul liberated. This may seem fanciful, but it is important to realize that that is what is being aimed at.

HARNESSING THE CHATTERING MIND

Controlling your breathing will have a direct effect on your mental activity. We know we need to approach the daily problems of life calmly if we are to cope with them properly. Try to practice the following two or three times a day, whether you feel stressed or not:

■ Sit comfortably erect.

■ Sit quietly, eyes closed, for two or three minutes.

■ Listen to your breathing and slow it down gradually.

■ Stressful issues can start to be seen in a proper perspective.

■ Stick to the same times each day. Discipline and routine are important here.

■ In due course, this exercise will become a natural pattern and result in far greater feelings of control.

■ Do not be upset if you struggle at first—your mind needs exercising and training much like your body.

■ Pain and physical discomfort can also be controlled in this way.

■ In due course, it will become possible to achieve greater control over your breathing exercises, but do not rush it.

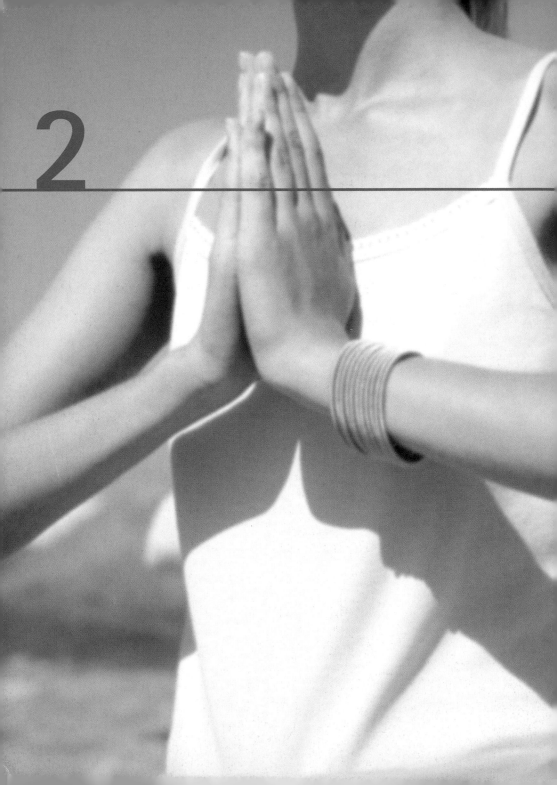

2

mind and body

In yoga, improved physical and mental health and well-being are achieved through the understanding that the mind and body are not separate entities but are, in fact, inextricably linked components of a unified whole. In practice, this means achieving balance and a clear mind through Hatha yoga or, as it can also be described, "cleaning the teeth" yoga. Additionally, this means becoming aware of, and gaining control of, how we breathe on a day-to-day basis and finding the correct posture in which to practice the asanas through three simple steps.

consciousness and the mind

Two of the great unsolved questions in life are "what is consciousness?" and "what is the mind?" More than 1,000 years ago, an early yoga sage declared: "What is pure consciousness? It is the life breath. And what is the life breath? It is pure consciousness."

This concept of a life breath, or life force, propelling reality (a reality the yogis believed was illusionary and termed *maya*) can be traced through almost all civilizations and the world's great religions. It is a belief, too, that is increasingly echoed in many of the theories advanced by contemporary particle physicists. In short, the more deeply we look into reality, the more we come to see that nothing is solid and that distinctions or boundaries between one thing and another, including the mind and the body, are essentially false.

At first, all of this may seem remote from—if not entirely irrelevant to—our everyday lives and the practice of yoga. But it is important to accept that the physical and the mental are in fact inextricably linked and do not exist on either side of a divide that cannot be crossed. This is key to understanding the constant interplay between mind and body that we can encourage through yoga to achieve greater mental and physical well-being.

A CLEAR MIND

One of the outstanding yogis of the twentieth century, Swami Sivananda, advised his followers to practice what he called "cleaning the teeth yoga" and "brushing the mat yoga." By this he meant that, however trivial the task we are performing, it should be carried out with total concentration. When we clean our teeth, the mind tends to wander. If, however, we concentrate on the job at hand, we will not only do it much better, but we begin to get into the habit of doing one thing at a time and not jumbling up our thoughts and actions. Thus the beneficial effects of these activities goes well beyond the activities themselves.

how yoga trains the mind

While the progressive development of yoga in our lives is likely to be centered on group and individual practice of the asanas, these can occupy only a small part of our average day. As has been stated in previous chapters, sages and scientists alike agree that thoughts, reactions, and emotions are communicated throughout the body, right down to the cellular level, either supporting the immune process or damaging it, according to the impulses that are radiated.

It quickly becomes apparent, therefore, that a 24-hour-a-day approach is required if yoga is to help us improve the mind–body relationship and sustain our overall good health and peace of mind. This may seem a daunting prospect at the outset but it will eventually become immensely rewarding. It is through just such an integrated approach to the practice of yoga that many people have come to enjoy a transformed life.

concentration

Further, the 24-hour-a-day approach actively encourages us to concentrate on our actions as we perform them This means learning to give our attention to one thing at at a time. Through this, we can start to develop mental clarity, which in turn leads to greater understanding of the physical body and its role in life.

Though this seems a simple idea, it still requires focus and concentration to carry it through in everyday life so that we become aware, for instance, of our posture, how we stand, sit, or hold ourselves at the wheel of a car. With perseverance, we eventually find ourselves maintaining good posture wherever we are, holding our shoulders without tension, sitting and standing erect, and so on, without having to think about it.

the yoga of balance

The approach to yoga most commonly practiced is called Hatha yoga, which is itself an aspect of Classical yoga. Some people talk of this as physical yoga, but that is not correct. We should regard it as yoga that, while it involves the body, also involves the mind and spirit. *Ha* and *tha* (pronounced "ta") are symbols for the sun and the moon. (The actual words in Sanskrit are *surya* and *chandra*.) This establishes it as the yoga of balance—balance between the various aspects that make up our lives.

In one sense, therefore, "brushing the teeth" yoga is Hatha yoga, for the physical action is linked with mental concentration and its purpose. While the act of brushing the teeth will have

some effect on the arm muscles, this is only a small part of the overall effect. The same idea applies to the asanas; the physical movements are pointless unless they are accompanied by mental concentration. In fact, many contemporary attitudes are revealed in the manner in which we perform asanas. Some people complete a yoga position carefully right to the end, while others leave it unfinished with their minds already on the next one. While the first example shows determination and conscientiousness, the second example is a sign of a confused life and the inability to cope with challenges. The mental discipline that yoga brings can help us clear up this confusion.

THE LIFE FORCE IN US

From time to time we should remind ourselves of the age-old wisdom and declare, "I am not a body." We exist in a body, but this can best be thought of as the mobile caravan of our lives. Remember that, with the exception of millions of brain cells, your body is changing all the time. You are constantly becoming a new person in the physical sense. However, the real "I"—the consciousness and the mind—remains stable.

What we call it—soul, spirit, or whatever else—does not matter. The real "I" in this human existence is personified by the life force that has been known to civilizations right across the world and has been depicted in art as diverse as Christian iconography, which often shows holy figures surrounded by auras, to Aboriginal wall paintings, which depict figures glowing.

YOGA AND THE BRAIN

Thanks to scientific tests in which the brain's electrical impulses have been recorded, it has been possible to examine the effects of yoga on brain function, especially its role in quieting the mind.

These all show that the combination of peaceful mental concentration, slow, rhythmical breathing, and controlled movement are linked with the brain waves moving from a state of agitation to one of balance and calm.

breathing

While Classical yoga specifies that *pranayama* (breathing) comes after the asana (see p. 7), it is important for us to remember that this code of practice was developed in a very different civilization from our own. The great majority of early disciples lived in mountainous regions, where the air was unpolluted, their posture was better, and the natural inborn breath was far easier to maintain. Today, young children walk and breathe naturally, but the detrimental aspects of modern life—poor body awareness, inappropriately designed environments, heavy pollution, increasing stress—all begin to take their toll quite early. Nevertheless, gaining day-to-day control over breathing is essential.

breathing and posture

Pranayama naturally links with the asanas. As we have seen, the asana as we know it today grew out of the sitting position for mind control and meditation. This involves having an erect spine, not, you will note, a straight one. The spine has natural curves and an erect posture balances these. It also enables the rib cage to

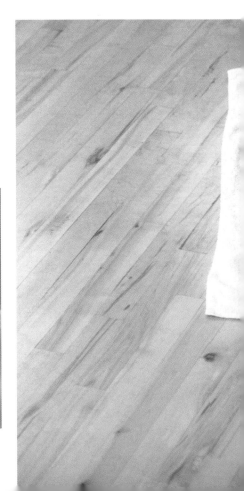

THE UNIQUENESS OF HOW WE BREATHE

Most of us give little or no thought to how we breathe. It comes automatically, and we know it is necessary to keep us alive, but that is about all. However, our bodies operate on two systems—the voluntary and the automatic. Usually these are separate, but our breathing is unique in that we can voluntarily modify how we breathe, as well as have it done automatically. Our ability to influence how we breathe is very important since it is a key way of stilling our minds.

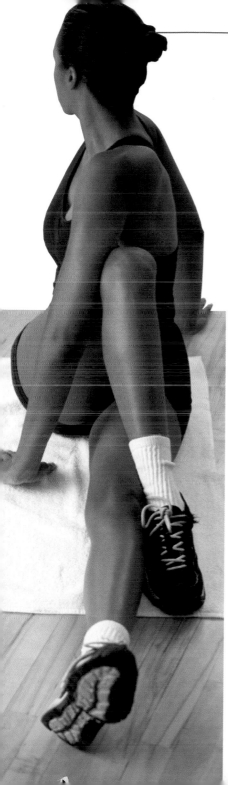

function naturally and the heart and diaphragm to move effectively. Finally, it ensures the correct interplay between the muscles of the trunk.

Using the head to carry things still persists in many parts of the world, especially in India, but in the West we have totally lost the art. We find it amusing when we see pictures of trainee models walking with books on their heads to maintain the right poise. Yet having your head and shoulders sagging forward impairs natural breathing, as does thrusting them back.

Yoga movements will encourage a return to effective posture, but we need to realize that it is important at all times, not just when carrying out the asanas, in order to make the most effective use of our lives.

Regular performance of the asanas in combination with controlled breathing will help concentrate the mind for a sustained meditation practice.

breathing and the asanas

Every yoga asana involves the breath. As a general rule, every movement made with exertion, however controlled, is performed on an in-breath and every relaxing movement on an out-breath. Where a pose is held, the breathing continues evenly and to the depth that is adequate for the exertion involved.

Performing postures regularly with the right attention to breathing will enhance everyday breathing naturally, but we should not just rely on that. As already mentioned, yoga is essentially an all-day, everyday activity, constantly developing the control over our own lives.

breathing awareness

Once you have checked that your posture is comfortably correct, you can take the first step in *pranayama*: learning to listen to your breathing. Just sit on a sensible chair—or on the floor—put your hands in your lap, close your eyes, and listen to your breathing. Do not interfere with it; simply observe it. In the normal way, it should be rather slow, even, and wholly unforced. It will, of course, change according to circumstances. If you do something physically demanding, it automatically deepens to enhance oxygen intake and circulation. If you are still, it will slow and be less deep—though not shallow.

basic breathing techniques

The processes of *pranayama* are varied and range from the simple to the comparatively complex. In the first stages of yoga practice, it is best to keep to the basic techniques of relaxed breathing and deep breathing, outlined in the section below. Both forms can be practiced in yoga sessions and it is also beneficial to use them from time to time throughout the day. Their importance cannot be overestimated.

When you have practiced the basic breathing and feel able to move on to the next stage, specific techniques can then be introduced. It is important to remember, however, to start slowly and perservere—there are no quick fixes. Both body and mind respond to calm persistence, but will react against being forced to do something they are not able to do.

relaxed breathing

Start by bringing your awareness to the breathing as described above. If you are in a reasonably peaceful state, you will find it is slow, quite rhythmical, and perfectly natural. The mind and body will be working together to create tranquility.

At first you may notice some problems; if your breathing doesn't slow, or feels uneven or forced in any way, then gently take control. Usually, we take between 14 and 16 breaths each minute. When we relax the breathing, this slows down to around six. If you have difficulty calming your breathing to this level, try counting to five as you breathe in and six to 10 as

FINDING THE CORRECT POSTURE

1 A simple way of checking how you normally use your body is to stand with your back to a wall, your heels about 1/2 in. (1 cm) from the wall itself, and your buttocks and shoulders touching it.

2 Then, using your thumb and forefinger as a measuring gauge, see how far the back of your head is from the wall. It should be the same distance as your heels.

3 Now walk round the room and try again. You will quickly establish whether or not you have maintained the natural stance.

TAKE A DEEP BREATH

It is essential to remember that our automatic breathing responds to and supports our emotions. In other words, if we are nervous, it will consolidate our nervousness, or, if we are angry, it will promote our anger. This is why, when people express strong emotion, they are often advised to take a few deep breaths to break the cycle. From this we can see how important it is that we can influence our own lives and reactions, based on our ability to change our breathing patterns voluntarily.

you breathe out. Or use a watch or clock with a second hand and time each breath—10 seconds for each inhalation and exhalation—until you feel it coming easily.

It is also advisable to spend a few minutes breathing deeply, using the lungs to full capacity. Again sitting correctly, first breathe out and then breathe in slowly and evenly, feeling the chest expand. Do not allow the abdomen to billow out; instead, keep the muscles there under control as the diaphragm lowers when the breath fills the lungs. This ensures equal pressure in both the chest and the abdomen, which generates the force on which body energy depends. A number of sessions will be necessary to transform old and constricting breathing patterns, but even a few breaths taken in this manner will recharge the body and clear the mind.

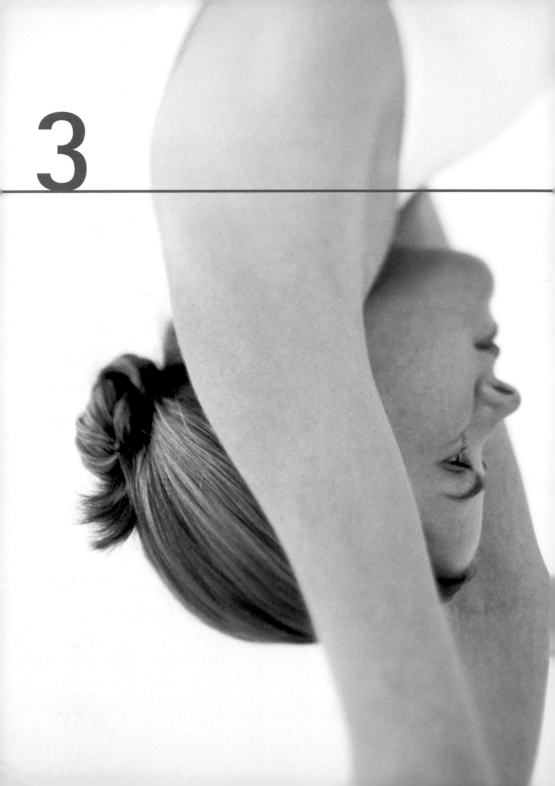

3

before you start

Before you start your yoga practice, it is good to be clear on the fundamental approach you should take and attend to some basic practicalities, such as clothes and equipment, as well as choosing an instructor who is right for you. Yoga should be performed in a state of relaxation and composure. This means deciding on a place and time that will allow you to practice daily without difficulty and which won't involve rushing to get to class, leaving no time to unwind, or missing sessions altogether. This section also includes a number of guidelines on general care and basic precautions as well as the six key steps that can be applied to each of the asanas.

getting started

We have already established that yoga is a complete approach to life and that it has a role to play in all our activities. All life, therefore, is a preparation for yoga, and yoga is a preparation for all life. However, what is commonly called the yoga session does need a special degree of preparation, whether it is performed in a group or alone.

when to practice yoga

Because digestion makes considerable demands on our bodies, no session of yoga asanas should be undertaken for at least 90 minutes after a snack, or two hours after a heavier meal. You should never rush into yoga and, therefore, however rushed life may be, make every attempt to allow sufficient time to get to the class venue and to relax and unwind before the session starts. Your instructor will allow adequate time for your consciousness to return to the concerns of the everyday world. Both group and individual sessions should mix physical activity with relaxation techniques, not only at the beginning and the end, but also at suitable intervals during the session itself.

personal yoga sessions

For many people the best time for a home session will be the early morning. Where practicable, it is worthwhile to have a very brief program before going to bed, with the emphasis on calming the mind, breathing slowly and rhythmically, and stretching gently.

When working at home, do all you can to avoid interruptions. Rather than taking the approach of rushing in and fixing things as we do in the outer world, enter your inner world through the techniques of preparation and relaxation.

An additional factor when working at home is that the responsibility for a balanced program is in your own hands. Asanas involve gentle stretching with no sharp tugging at unprepared muscles or joints. The back appreciates equal movement in all directions: so many back conditions could be prevented if the spine was kept sensibly flexible.

CHOOSING AN INSTRUCTOR

Sessions can either be in a group class, or as a one-on-one.
■ For group sessions, it is important to find the right teacher. This can be a matter of trial and error. It is helpful for the instructor to hold an appropriate training certificate, but the process is as much a matter of empathy as technical training. If possible, therefore, you should try to find the opportunity for a trial session or two before committing yourself. As in the choice of spiritual adviser, or doctor, the relationship is extremely important.
■ During one-on-one sessions, your instructor will be necessarily able to devote more time to you and explore issues that are not always possible in a group class. It is especially important that you have a good relationship with your instructor before doing one-on-one sessions.

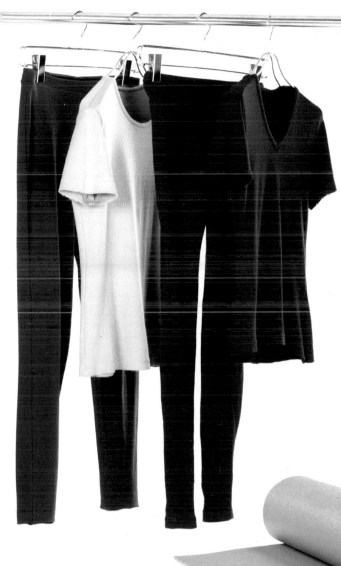

CLOTHING AND EQUIPMENT

Clothing should be loose enough not to restrict movement or blood flow at any point, but not so loose as to make you trip over yourself. You can wear anything from a sweatsuit, to sportswear, to loose pants and a comfortable T-shirt.

Your feet should be bare for yoga practice, as socks or panty hose can slip on mats and floors.

Remove tightly strapped watches and any awkward jewelry.

Don't wear a restrictive belt. Tie back any long hair.

Buy or borrow a yoga mat, big enough for you to stretch out on fully, and thick enough to protect your spine against the floor. It should also give a good grip for your feet.

Use a comfortably upright chair when you start practicing your breathing and meditation.

Comfortable clothing and a yoga mat are all you need to start your asana practice.

a unique activity

When you begin to practice Hatha yoga (the physically active component of yoga), you may be surprised to find that it is unlike any other form of sport or exercise. Its uniqueness makes it special.

It seems extraordinary that a philosophy and practice with such an ancient history should have total and vital relevance to modern life; the passing of time has not diminished its value to the current generation.

One of the most important points to remember is that there is no aspect of competition, either with others or even with yourself—your own assessment of your ability at this moment. Make the wonderful, liberating expression "Be here now" your key phrase.

So, observations such as "Have I managed to stretch farther than I did last week?" and "My classmates do it much better than I do" are not important in any way.

Proceed through your practice routine in a peaceful frame of mind, detached from both self-criticism and self-praise, focused on the quiet but

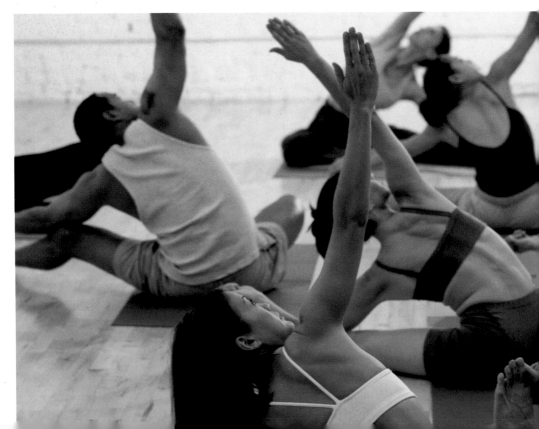

powerful interaction of your mind, body, and breath. The more familiar you become with the asanas you will learn, the greater will be your ability to detach yourself from analyzing and concentrating on what your body is doing so that even a physical movement becomes a meditative experience.

The terms "intermediate," "advanced," and "expert" do not have a place in yoga practice. As we have seen, this is because there is no competition in yoga and no concept

STILLNESS

1 Both a person new to yoga and a person who has been studying yoga for many years will be able to practice the same asanas and gain benefit in the same way.

2 In fact, someone who can sit perfectly still in a contemplative way may be practicing yoga at a much deeper level than someone who is only capable of performing the physical movements of the asanas.

3 So don't forget that we only use the physical practice as a means to being able to sit still. Stillness is, paradoxically, the essence of Hatha yoga.

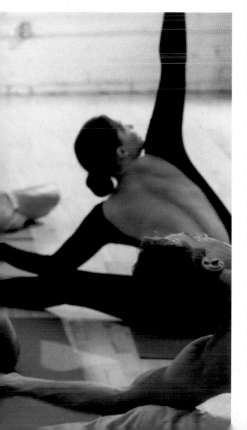

of forced progress or end-gaining. This is a simple idea but one that can be hard to keep at the forefront of our minds, since it runs contrary to the competitive nature of society, where people often feel that unless they are putting all their energy into getting ahead then they will be left behind. This energy often shows itself as the fear of failure, which is a powerful motivating tool, but one which can have disasterous consequences on our health when we find we cannot cope under such strain. And, yes, a lot of it is indeed self-inflicted (see p. 90 for the subject of self-responsibility).

starting your session

Ideally, your practice area should be in a quiet room with no distractions of any kind, either from members of the family or the telephone. However, if you find this difficult, do your best to find some space for yourself at a time when the likelihood of interruption is minimal. Have your room at a comfortable temperature, neither too hot nor too cold. It is a good idea to use a non-slip mat, even though your room may be carpeted; it helps to define your working space and will prevent accidental slipping.

Begin by lying on the floor in the pose of *Savasana* (see p. 79). The intention is not to achieve a state of deep relaxation at this stage, simply to relax the body before you begin, compose your thoughts and center yourself mentally by being aware of any current problems you may have

The asanas were originally meant to be held in the extreme position for some time in order that the mind become still and meditative. You may find this challenging at first, so do not continue to hold any position which begins to cause discomfort.

At the end of your chosen routine, lie down once again in *Savasana* (p. 79), taking care to position your body correctly on your mat.

This time the length of your relaxation should be longer than at the start—around 15 minutes is ideal. However, the actual time is not important—the depth and quality of the relaxation is.

The following steps can be applied to each asana:

1 relax

Relax and gradually become aware of your breathing.

2 visualize

Visualize the posture you are going to perform and focus your awareness on those parts of the body that you intend to move or stretch.

3 ability

Perform the asana to the best of your ability, linking the movements to your breathing and not allowing your thoughts to wander.

4 control

Come out of the asana in a controlled, unhurried manner and return to the starting position.

5 focus

Relax, focusing once again on your breathing.

6 balance

If the posture is one that needs to be practiced to both left and right, take a slow balancing breath before repeating the movement on the second side.

GENERAL CARE AND PRECAUTIONS

POINTS TO REMEMBER:

1 Consult your doctor before starting a yoga course, particularly if you have recently had an illness, surgery, or injury.

2 Work within your own capabilities and be aware of any limitations or health problems you may have. Even a minor illness, such as a cold, will temporarily affect your body's ability to work.

3 Do not ignore signals of discomfort from your body. As a general rule, pain means STOP. Your muscles may feel tight at first, and your back stiff, but gentle, sensible perseverance will help you become more supple and flexible.

4 Consult your doctor before starting a yoga course if you are pregnant. However, it is usually safe to practice during a normal pregnancy. Toward the end of your pregnancy, postures that compress or fully stretch the abdomen will not be possible, but gentle stretches for the back and flexibility exercises for the legs and pelvis will be beneficial. In addition, there are special yoga courses available for pregnant women.

5 Inverted postures should be avoided by those with high blood pressure. If you feel dizzy at any time, particularly in forward bending, return to the upright position.

6 Do not raise or lower straight legs while lying supine on the floor. Always bend your knees first to prevent strain on your back.

7 Never force or strain; remember to relax into each movement.

8 If you find your back is uncomfortable when lying on the floor with your legs extended, most postures, including *Savasana*, can be adapted by performing them with your knees bent.

9 Practice regularly—little and often is best. Three 20-minute sessions a week is a good starting point.

10 Avoid pushing yourself too hard. As we have said, yoga is never a competition with anyone or anything, not even with your own previous efforts.

11 Relax at the end of a session. Keep a blanket and socks handy to stay warm.

12 Always be aware of your breathing, synchronizing the physical movements to the breath and not the other way round.

and putting them aside for the duration of the session.

A period of five minutes is often sufficient, but, if you are feeling restless or agitated, wait until you feel more balanced before you start to move and stretch. The same applies, of course, to feeling excessively excited or on a "high."

Practice your asanas in a calm, relaxed state of mind, totally focused on yourself and your body.

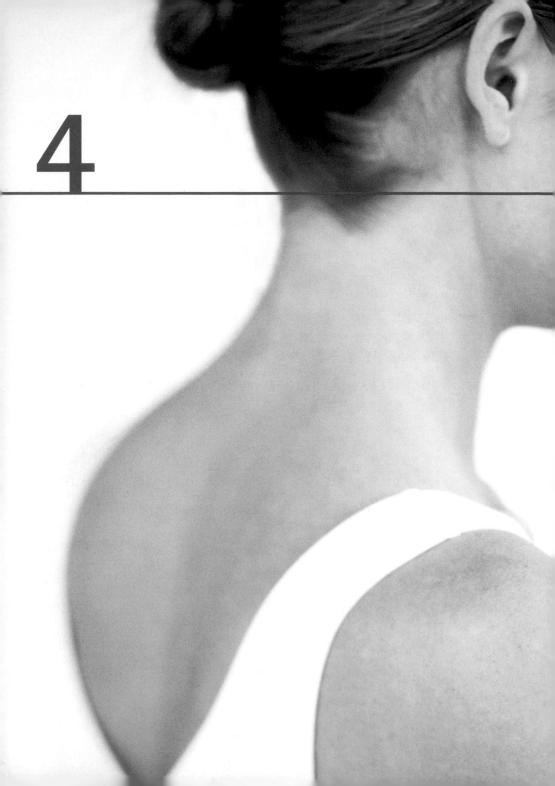

4

the asanas

The following section comprises 33 fully
illustrated asanas with step-by-step captions
and a clear explanation of the benefits of each
move. The order of the asanas offers a logical
sequence to follow, but can be adapted in any
way to suit your own requirements. These asanas
range from the Full Body Stretch to the Savasana,
with classic positions such as the Cow's Head, Cat,
Downward Dog, Child, Camel, Boat, Tree, Warrior,
and many more in between.

There is also, throughout, additional information
on the kinds of sensations and feelings that you may
be experiencing with individual moves, along with
hints and tips on how you can adapt your technique
or approach should you experience any initial
difficulty, discomfort, or stiffness.

the asanas

The first two asanas are stretches that provide a wonderful way to start your session. They tone muscles, loosen joints, and improve breathing. The Knee Squeeze improves flexibility in the hips and circulation in the abdominal organs.

FULL BODY STRETCH

1

Lie on your back, legs extended, arms by your sides. Lengthen the back of your neck by keeping your chin tucked in, and relax your body.

Inhale and raise both arms over your head until they touch the floor behind you.

If this is too difficult or your shoulders are too stiff at first, place a cushion or a folded blanket on the floor behind your head for your arms to rest on.

LYING SIDE STRETCH

2

Lie on your back, your legs extended, your arms by your sides, and your hands touching your legs.

Keeping your bottom and legs still, begin to move your head and shoulders to the right while facing the ceiling. Allow your hands to move with your body.

Relax into the position and be aware of the left side of your body stretching and your left lung expanding. Hold for about 10 breaths.

KNEE SQUEEZE

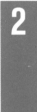

Lie on your back with your legs extended. Bring your left knee toward your chest and clasp it with both hands.

If this feels uncomfortable, place your hands on the back of your thigh underneath your knee instead.

Check that the whole of your leg feels relaxed from your hip to your foot. This also applies to your right leg.

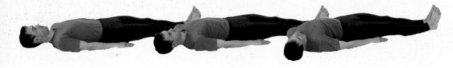

how's it going?

Your whole body will tingle with a renewed flow of energy as you perform the first two asanas. As you begin to stretch, imagine your body opening and extending like a flower opening its petals to the morning sunshine. If your muscles are stiff at first, don't worry; just do the best you can. The Knee Squeeze also promotes energy flow and circulation as well as improving suppleness in the hips and legs.

≜ how's it going?

As you inhale, stretch your right arm and right leg strongly, keeping your left arm and left leg relaxed. Feel the stretch from your fingertips to your heels.

Release the stretch as you exhale, then repeat the stretch three times. Repeat with the left arm and left leg, allowing the right side to relax

Finally, stretch both arms and legs together, trying not to hollow the back too much. Repeat three times. As you exhale, bring both arms back to your sides and relax.

If you feel comfortable with this position, bend your left elbow and place it under your head, softening your shoulder muscles. Hold for five breaths.

To increase the stretch, cross your left ankle over your right ankle. Hold for five breaths.

Return to the center position and repeat to the right.

As you exhale, gently draw your knee as close as you can to your chest. Try to keep the back of your right knee touching the floor.

As you inhale, release the stretch but keep hold of your knee. Repeat the squeeze three times more.

Release your left knee and place your leg back on the floor. Repeat the exercise, holding your right knee.

▶▶

4-5

the asanas continued

In our everyday lives, we rarely use the full range of movement in our hips. The Hip Loosener provides a way of opening up the muscles and joints in this area while the Pelvic Tilt works gently on the back to improve flexibility.

HIP LOOSENER

4

Lie on your back with your legs extended and your arms a little way out from your sides.

Draw your knees up, keeping your feet together. With your left leg still, allow your right knee to fall outward toward the floor. Hold for five breaths, allowing your hip to relax a little more with each exhalation.

Bring your knee upright again, then repeat on your left knee. You may find that one knee does not go down as far as the other. If this is the case, hold the position longer on the less flexible side to encourage more movement in the stiffer hip.

PELVIC TILT

5

Lie on your back with your knees bent, your feet hip-width apart, and your arms by your sides with the palms downward. Feel the whole of your spine in contact with the floor and tuck your chin in.

As you inhale, lift your stomach upward to create a small hollow under your lower back, but keep your bottom on the floor. You can check this by sliding one hand under your back at waist level.

As you exhale, reverse the movement by making your spine convex. Push your lower back into the floor, tightening your abdominal muscles and curling your tail under strongly.

how's it going?

As we grow older, the wonderful range of movement and suppleness that we enjoyed as children decreases and our joints naturally become stiffer and the movement more restricted. Asanas such as the Hip Loosener redress this, encouraging our bodies to regain that child-like suppleness. The Pelvic Tilt is a gentle asana, because your back is completely supported. This means it can be practiced safely by anyone—even those with back problems can use this technique to ease aches and pains.

⏶ how's it going?

Exhale as you let both knees fall outward at the same time. They will not go as far this time but use your exhalation to help relax your inner leg muscles. Check that your back does not arch too much.

Inhale and raise both arms behind your head and stretch strongly. Exhale as you soften your elbows but keep your arms behind your head.

Repeat the arm stretch three times, maintaining the same leg position. Finally, return your arms to your sides and bring both knees up again.

Do not jerk your back but make the movement slow and smooth so that the time it takes to change from one position to the other lasts the whole of the breath.

Repeat this movement 10 times, allowing this rocking motion to follow the natural flow of your breathing.

At first you may not feel much happening, but, as you progress, you will be surprised at how much more flexible your spine will become.

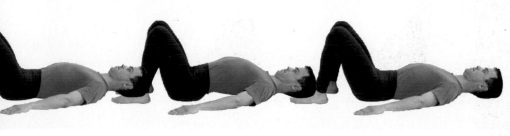

▶▶

6-7

the asanas continued

The Bridge stretches the muscles in the legs and hips, and opens the chest to aid deeper breathing, while the Lying Spinal Twist improves flexibility in the back and increases energy flow to the spine and abdominal organs.

BRIDGE

6

Lie on your back with your knees bent, your feet hip-width apart, and your arms by your sides, palms downward. Gently squeeze your shoulder blades together to open your chest and check that your chin is tucked in.

It is important to place your feet in the correct position—your heels must be directly under your knees. As you exhale, curl your tail under, flattening your back against the floor.

Inhale and, starting from the base of the spine, begin to lift your back from the floor as far as you can, supporting your weight on your shoulders, arms, and feet.

LYING SPINAL TWIST

7

Lie down on your back with your knees drawn up, your feet together and flat on the floor, and your arms by your sides.

As you inhale, move both arms out to shoulder level with your arms straight and the palms of your hands turned downward, in contact with the floor.

As you exhale, allow both knees to fall slowly to the left, keeping them together. See how far down they will go.

how's it going?

The Bridge is more demanding physically than the Pelvic Tilt, but still offers a safe and useful way to move the spine. If you have a serious back problem, such as chronic inflammation or a damaged disc, do not practice the Lying Spinal Twist. However, If your back is healthy, your spine will greatly benefit from this asana. The type of motion involved is called a torsion-type movement, where one end of the spine is held still, while the other end is twisted around.

⬆ how's it going?

Imagine that you are peeling your spine off the floor, one vertebra at a time as you lift up. Hold this position for three breaths.

Exhale and replace your back on the floor, vertebra by vertebra.

Finish by curling your tail under strongly, as in the starting position. Repeat the whole movement three times.

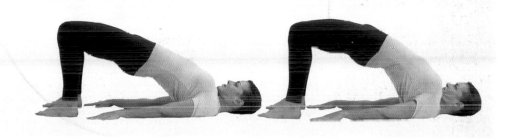

If they will not reach the ground, try placing a cushion or foam block under your knees for extra support.

Turn your head to the right, taking it as far as you can. Hold for 10 breaths, feeling your back relaxing with each exhalation, and keeping your left shoulder in contact with the floor.

Return to the center position as you inhale, and then repeat the stretch, this time taking your knees to the right and turning your head to the left.

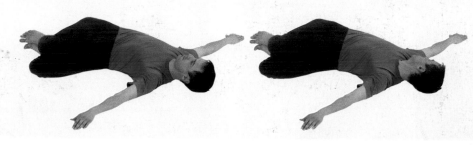

▶▶

8-9

the asanas continued

The Neck Stretches and Cow's Head will gently loosen your neck and upper back and counteract tightness in the shoulders often caused by stress.

NECK STRETCHES

8

Sit comfortably with your back straight.

Exhale as you slowly rotate your head so that you are looking over your right shoulder.

Hold this position for three breaths, relaxing into it. Keep your shoulders relaxed and your head upright.

COW'S HEAD

9

Sit upright. If you can, cross your right leg over your left, so the tops of your feet are on the floor.

If you cannot do this, simply sit comfortably on the floor or on a chair.

Raise your right arm, stretch it, then drop your right hand to touch the back of your neck.

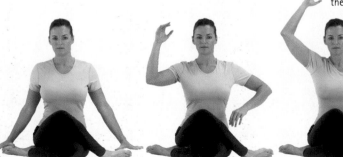

how's it going?

A flexible neck, shoulders, and upper back are very important in all aspects of our daily routine, including sleeping. If your body is not relaxed and comfortable lying in bed, your sleep will be shallow and interrupted. If you cannot join your hands in the Cow's Head, hold a scarf or belt in your upper hand and take hold of it with your lower hand. It is much more effective to use this method than to encourage strain and tension by attempting something that is beyond your present capabilities.

▲ how's it going?

Inhale as you slowly return to the center position. Repeat to the left side.

Exhale as you lower your chin to your chest, feeling the stretch in your neck and upper back muscles. Hold for three breaths.

Inhale as you raise your head to the normal position.

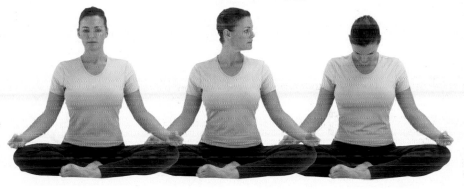

Take your left arm behind your back, bending the elbow upward, and see if you can clasp your hands together.

Hold, breathing evenly and relaxing your shoulders. Feel the stretch in the back of your right arm.

Hold for five breaths, keeping your back upright and your chest open. Then repeat on the other side.

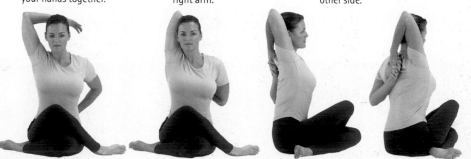

▶▶

10-11

the asanas continued

In addition to working on the spine, the Cat helps to deepen and balance the breathing while the Downward Dog strengthens the arms and shoulders and stretches the back.

CAT

10 Start on your hands and knees with your feet relaxed. Check that your hands are directly under your shoulders and your knees are under your hips.

Your hands should be facing forward with the fingers gently spread. Start off with your back straight and your neck in line with your spine so that you are looking at the floor.

As you inhale, hollow your back by relaxing your stomach downward and lifting your head up. Start the movement at your tail and let it flow up your spine in a wave-like motion.

DOWNWARD DOG

11 Take up the Cat position (above) on your hands and knees, spreading your fingers a little on the floor.

As you exhale, move your spine into the upward position and turn your toes under.

Inhale as you lift your hips up as high as you can, taking your knees off the floor. Start to straighten your legs and make them very strong.

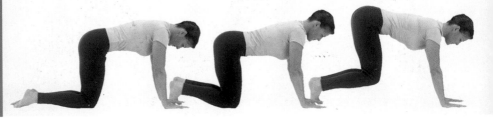

how's it going?

Like the Pelvic Tilt, the Cat is a safe and simple method of exercising the spine and improving suppleness—you only have to observe a cat for a few moments to marvel at the superb flexibility of its body. In addition, it also enhances the natural rhythm of the breath. You may find the Downward Dog challenging to start with. Its strengthening qualities for the upper body makes it a useful preparation for the more advanced Headstand.

▲ how's it going?

As you exhale, lift your back upward and allow your head to hang down between your arms. Continue this up-and-down movement of your back, synchronizing it with your breathing.

Do not bend your elbows—keep them straight, with your arms strong. Also, try not to sway to and fro—your arms and legs should hardly move. All motion should take place in the spine, head, and neck.

Make both your breathing and your movements as slow as you can. As you continue to practice you will be aware that you are able to take deeper breaths and achieve more flexibility in your spine.

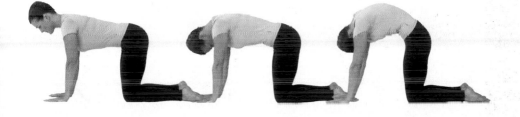

Exhale as you take your body weight backward, still supporting yourself on your toes, and stretch your arms.

Gently lower your heels toward the floor, keeping your back as straight as possible and taking your head down between your arms to form a "V" shape.

To increase the stretch, bend your right knee, feeling an extra stretch in your left leg. Hold for three breaths, and repeat with your left leg. Then straighten both legs, hold, and come down.

▶▶

12-13

the asanas continued

Like the Downward Dog, the Upward Dog is a powerful pose and has similar strengthening qualities in the upper body. It also opens the chest. The Child, meanwhile, allows the spine to bend the other way, opening it up.

UPWARD DOG

12

From the Downward Dog position, inhale as you lift your head and bring your body weight forward over your arms.

Keeping your arms very strong, start to lower your pelvis toward the floor. You may find you need to move your feet back a little.

As you exhale, keep your awareness in your back and slowly lower your pelvis as far as you can into the "plank" position.

CHILD

13

Sit on your heels with your knees bent, your arms by your sides, and your head facing forward. Keeping your bottom in contact with your heels, slowly bend forward, keeping your back straight and your head in line with your spine.

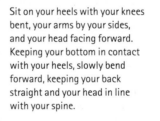

how's it going?

The Upward Dog follows the Downward Dog very well, but it is not advised for those with back or arm problems. To help you become used to the stretches in these areas, as well as the back and legs, you can bend your knees a little, with your heels off the floor. If you have a large mirror, you can practice the Dog in front of it and see how you are getting on. The Child is a good counter-pose to the very powerful Upward Dog, but an older person may find it difficult. If you find it too uncomfortable at this stage, come back to it later on as you improve in your practice.

▲ how's it going?

As you lower yourself farther, you will create a concave curve in your spine. Do not touch the floor with your stomach or thighs.

Keep your head up and your chest forward as you stretch strongly upward, breathing slowly for five breaths.

To come out, push up into the Downward Dog before bringing your knees back to the floor.

As your forehead moves down, take your hands back to rest by your feet, palms facing upward.

A useful alternative if you cannot reach the floor with your head is to move your hands out in front of you, make two fists, place one fist on top of the other, the sides your hands facing downward, and rest your forehead on the top fist.

If you find sitting on your heels difficult, lie down on your back instead with your knees bent in order to gain the same benefits of recovery and relaxation.

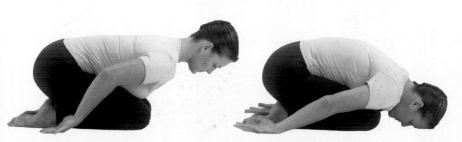

▶▶

14-15

the asanas continued

The Sitting Forward Bend stretches the back and the backs of the legs, while the Sitting Spinal Twist, like the Lying Spinal Twist (see pp. 50–51), improves flexibility in the back.

SITTING FORWARD BEND

14

Sit with your legs extended and your back upright. Place your hands under your buttocks and gently lift up and back to sit more on the front of the pelvis.

Inhale as you raise both arms out to the sides, then above your head, and stretch upward.

SITTING SPINAL TWIST

15

Sit upright, with your back straight and your legs extended in front of you.

Place your right foot on the floor on the outside of your left knee. If this feels forced or strained, place it on the inside of the left knee instead.

Hold your right knee firmly with your left hand or wrap your elbow around it.

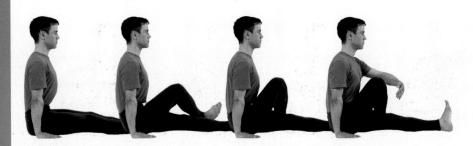

how's it going?

The need to relax into postures applies particularly to the Sitting Forward Bend. As you take your torso forward, relax into it, using the exhalation. If your back is stiff, sit on a small cushion in order to help tilt your pelvis forward. You can also bend your knees. The Sitting Spinal Twist is a little more demanding than the Lying version. Approach it in stages so that you feel happy and comfortable in the first stage before you move on to the next. In all sitting twists, it is important that your back remains dynamically upright—do not let it hunch or curl forward.

⏶ how's it going?

Keeping your head up, exhale as you bend forward with your back straight, reaching as far as you can toward your feet.

Touch your hands lightly to the furthest part of your legs you can reach without straining. Hold for up to 10 breaths, breathing slowly, relaxing your head and neck, and checking that your elbows and shoulders are soft.

On each inhalation, see if you can stretch a little farther forward; on each exhalation relax farther down. Return to the upright position on an inhalation, by either raising your arms or sliding your hands up your legs.

Extend your right arm forward at shoulder level and take it around to the right as far as you can, turning your head in the same direction.

Place your right hand on the floor behind you, lined up with the center of your body, fingers pointing backward. Inhale and hold the pose, lengthening your neck and straightening your spine.

As you exhale, see if you can twist around a little farther, looking over your right shoulder. Hold for five breaths. Then return to the center position and repeat on the other side.

16-17

the asanas continued

The Kneeling Back Bend and the Camel are both back bends that involve a stretching and opening of the front of the body, expanding the chest.

KNEELING BACK BEND

16

Sit on your heels. Take your hands back behind you, keeping your fingers pointing forward. Create a bend in the spine by arching your body and allowing your head to tilt back. Make sure your elbows remain straight, with your arms strongly stretched, and push your breastbone forward. Hold for three breaths.

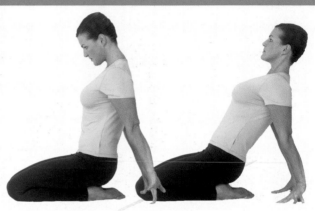

CAMEL

17

Kneel on the floor, knees hip-width apart and feet relaxed. Inhale as you put your hands on your hips. Exhale as you bend backward, allowing your head to tilt back. Gently press your elbows together to encourage the spine to bend and the chest to open; be sure to keep your hips pushed forward.

Hold for three breaths. Come up slowly and carefully, raising your head first.

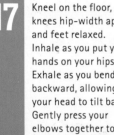

how's it going?

The Kneeling Back Bend and the Camel represent two ways of bending the spine backward, either as separate asanas or as a counterpose to a forward bend, such as the Sitting Forward Bend (pp. 58–59), which compresses the chest. By their nature, they involve some compression of the back. If you have a history of back pain or stiffness, you must approach them gently and slowly and stop immediately if you feel any pain.

⬆ how's it going?

This posture also offers a good stretch to the wrists and forearm muscles and can be used as an alternative to the Fish to follow the Shoulder Stand.

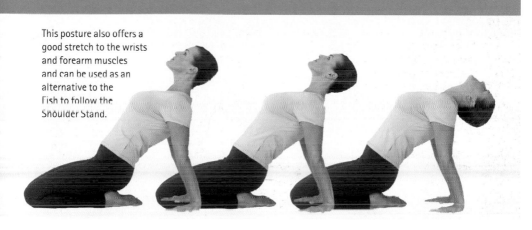

Then turn your toes under, place your hands on your heels one at a time, and repeat, holding for three breaths.

Remember to push your pelvis forward and keep your thighs in a vertical position.

Place the tops of your feet flat on the floor, place your hands on your heels, and hold for three breaths. This is a more testing back bend, so stop if you feel any discomfort.

▶▶

18-19

the asanas continued

The Boat and the Standing Knee Squeeze are both balance asanas. The Boat strengthens the muscles of the back, abdomen, and legs, while the Standing Knee Squeeze strengthens the legs and promotes flexibility in the hips.

BOAT

18

Sit with your knees bent and your feet on the floor. Check that you have space behind you in case you lose your balance and roll back. Clasp the backs of your thighs with your hands.

Sit forward on your pelvis by pulling up your lower back. Roll back on your buttocks enough to maintain a balanced position and lift your feet off the floor.

Keeping your back straight and your chin tucked in, slowly straighten your knees and start to raise your legs.

As you raise your legs to 45 degrees, hold the balance, breathing evenly.

Turn your palms downward and stretch your arms forward. Hold for up to five breaths.

If you feel stable, take your hands away from your legs and straighten your arms, parallel to the floor.

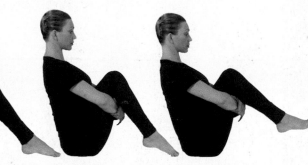

how's it going?

The Boat, as with all balance postures, demands concentration and you may find it challenging to start with. It is better to start practicing this posture with a rounded back until you feel confident enough to try it with a straight back. The Standing Knee Squeeze is also a balance posture and is the standing version of the Knee Squeeze (pp. 46–47). If you have knee problems, you may find it more comfortable to take hold of your lower thigh, underneath the knee, rather than the front of the shin as shown here.

⌃ how's it going?

STANDING KNEE SQUEEZE

19

Stand with your feet together, your arms by your sides. Inhale as you bend your right knee and raise it to waist height. Clasp it firmly with both hands.

Draw the knee up as far you can, relaxing your hip and supporting the weight of the leg with your hands. Keep your back straight and make sure you draw your knee toward your chest, rather than your chest toward your knee.

Maintain the balance, breathing steadily and calmly. Hold for five breaths. Release the leg and return to a standing position, then repeat with the other leg.

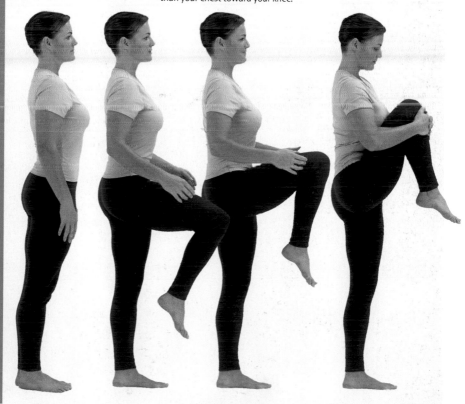

▸▸

20

the asanas continued

The Standing Balance stretches the front of the thighs and the arms, shoulders, and sides of the body. It also strengthens the legs.

STANDING BALANCE

20

Stand with your feet together, arms by your sides. Feel that your left leg is very strong and visualize energy flowing from your foot down into the floor.

Inhale and bend your right knee, taking your foot back behind you; hold it with your right hand.

Exhale as you draw your foot as close as you can to your bottom. Relax the whole leg from the hip to the toes, allowing your knee to drop toward the floor.

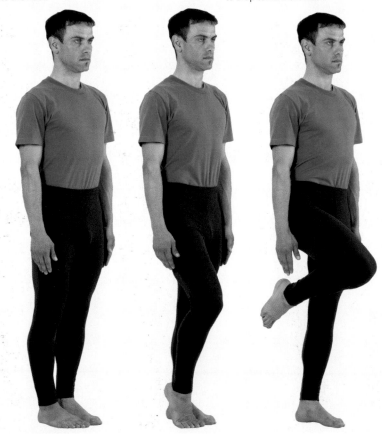

how's it going?

You will find that balancing postures are just as much a mental exercise as a physical one. Trying to balance on one leg when you are feeling agitated or distracted will result in you wobbling and swaying. So, as you stand in the starting position, first focus your mind on the calm, even flow of your breath; gaze at a spot on the floor just ahead of you and keep your awareness in your throat area. When you feel relaxed and in control, begin the asana.

☱ how's it going?

Inhale as you raise your left arm and stretch upward. Take your arm as close as you can to your ear. Extend the stretch to your fingertips.

Hold the position, breathing calmly for five breaths. Lower your arm, release your foot and repeat on the other side.

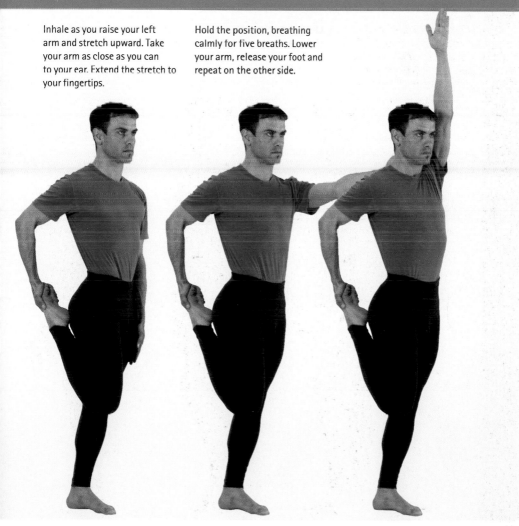

▶▶

the asanas continued

The Triangle is also performed standing, this time incorporating a side bend. It stretches and strengthens the sides of the body, hips, back, shoulders, and arms.

TRIANGLE

Stand with your feet apart (approximately the length of your inside leg). Turn out your left foot to 90 degrees and pivot on your right heel, bringing your toes inward. Check that your left heel is in line with your right instep.

Inhale as you raise both arms to shoulder level. Exhale as you bend your body to the left, taking your left hand down to touch your left leg and raising your right hand to the ceiling.

Turn your right hand so that your palm is facing forward, then turn your head to look up at the hand. If you have neck problems, do not turn your head too far. Hold this position, breathing evenly and slowly, for five breaths.

how's it going?

In this asana you will breathe more into one lung than the other, since one will be compressed by your body position. Come out of the pose carefully as you release your supporting hand to return to an upright position, inhaling deeply. The Triangle is essentially a side bend and care should be taken that your hips do not turn, making it a forward bend as well. You can check this by practicing against a wall and seeing that both shoulder blades touch the wall.

▲ how's it going?

Remember to actively reach upward with your right hand, stretching the right side of your body.

Return to an upright position as you inhale and lower your arms.

Then repeat the Triangle on the other side, not forgetting to begin by turning your feet to the right.

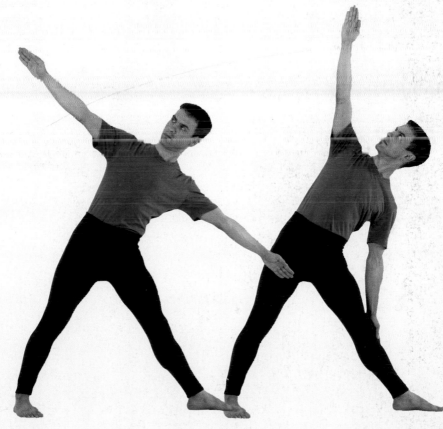

▶▶

22-23

the asanas continued

A s its name implies, the Warrior is a dynamic asana, generating energy and confidence from a position of grounded strength. The Tree tones the legs and opens the hips.

WARRIOR

22 Stand with your feet wide apart. Turn your right foot out to 90 degrees and the toes of your left foot inward. Bend your right knee to 90 degrees. Make your legs strong, keeping your weight on the outsides of your feet. Inhale as you raise both arms to shoulder level and stretch them strongly. Turn your head and look along your right arm. Hold the position for five breaths, keeping your torso straight. Come out of the posture by turning your head, straightening your legs and lowering your arms. Repeat on the other side.

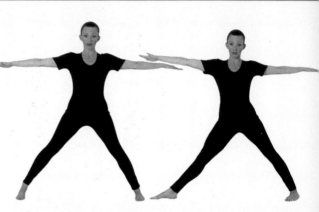

TREE

23 Stand with your feet together, and your hands together as if praying. Taking your weight on your right leg, place your left foot firmly against the inside of your right thigh, as high up the leg as you can. Check that your left knee is pointing out to the side. Breathe calmly. Then bring your hands to chest level, palms together. Hold for three breaths. As you inhale, stretch your arms above your head, palms together. Hold for three more breaths. Open your arms to shoulder width, palms facing each other. Hold for three deep breaths. Exhale as you come out of the pose, then repeat on your left leg.

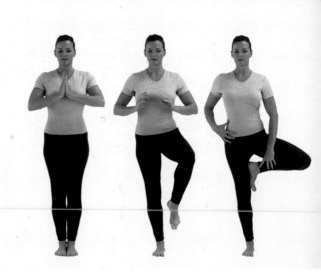

how's it going?

The Warrior can be very challenging but it is worthwhile persevering. The key is to place your feet wide enough apart to obtain the correct position for your legs. This may prove difficult at first. Remember that your heel must be directly under your knee on your bent leg. As you hold the pose, make your arms and legs very strong and breathe slowly and deeply. If the Tree is too difficult at first, you can place your foot against your right ankle with your toes touching the floor. Also, be cautious when practicing this asana if you have any knee or ankle problems.

▲ how's it going?

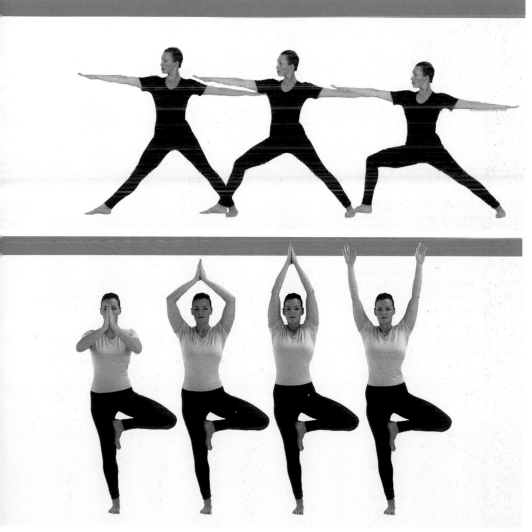

▶▶

24-25

the asanas continued

The Forward Bent Twist effectively stretches the legs, arms, and back as well as giving all the benefits of the twist. The Shoulder Stand is an inverted pose that strengthens the whole body and stimulates the circulatory and nervous systems.

FORWARD BENT TWIST

24 Stand with your legs wide apart and feet forward. Raise both arms to shoulder level and rotate your torso to the right as far as you can. Place the palm of your left hand on the floor midway between your feet. Leaving your left hand on the floor, inhale as you take your right arm outward and upward toward the ceiling, turning your head and upper body to the right.

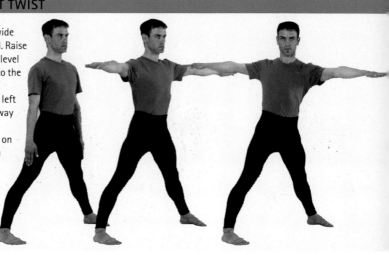

SHOULDER STAND

25 Lie on your back with your knees bent and your arms by your sides, palms down. Squeeze your shoulder blades together to ensure that your elbows will be as close together as possible when you lift up. Keep the back of your neck long by tucking your chin in.

Bend your knees and bring them toward your chest. Begin to extend your legs and take them over your head. At the same time, lift your buttocks and lower back off the floor and bring your hands to your lower back. Take your weight on your upper back and shoulders.

Bend your knees and make your back as straight as you can, checking that your elbows are close together. If you feel balanced and you have no discomfort in your neck, straighten your legs and extend them upward, keeping both hands on your back for support. Hold for as long as it is comfortable.

how's it going?

The Forward Bent Twist is the third of our twists and is done in a standing position. If you cannot touch the floor easily with your legs straight, place a chair in front of you and put your hands on the seat instead of on the floor. It is important to stay focused while getting into the Shoulder Stand. Do not swing your legs up, but keep control of the changes of position by using your muscles. This posture is not advised for women during their period or for those with neck problems, high blood pressure, or heart problems.

� how's it going?

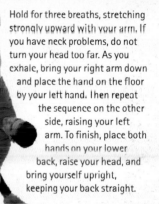

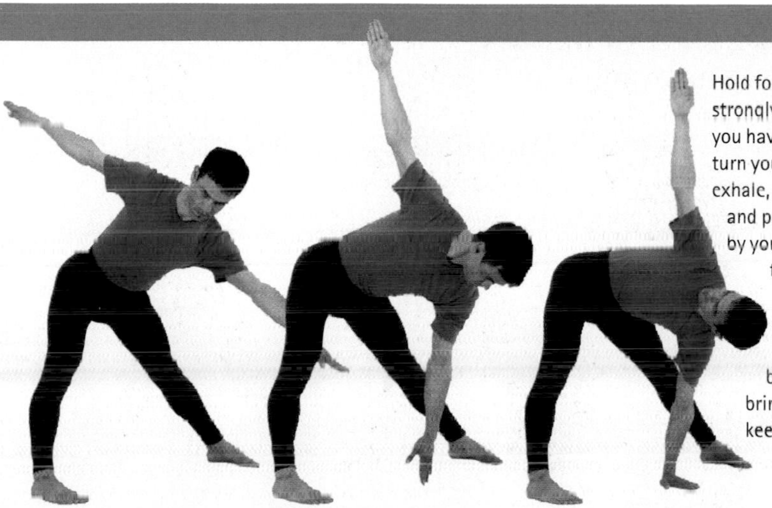

Hold for three breaths, stretching strongly upward with your arm. If you have neck problems, do not turn your head too far. As you exhale, bring your right arm down and place the hand on the floor by your left hand. Then repeat the sequence on the other side, raising your left arm. To finish, place both hands on your lower back, raise your head, and bring yourself upright, keeping your back straight.

To come out of the pose, bend your knees toward your face then straighten your legs as you extend them over your head. Place both hands on the floor, then slowly roll down with bent knees until you are lying on your back once more with your feet flat on the floor.

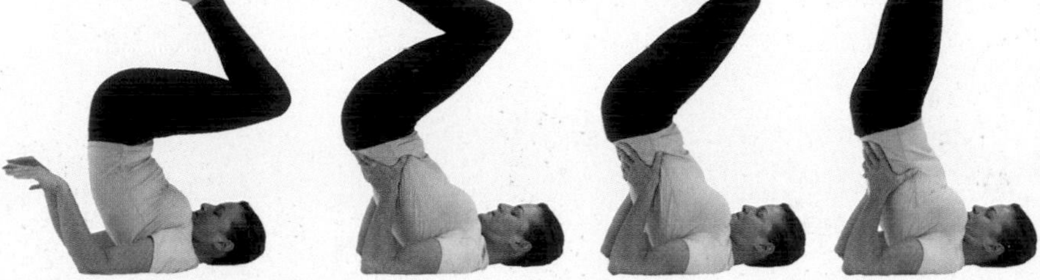

▶▶

26-27

the asanas continued

The Plough and the Fish follow the Shoulder Stand and complement its benefits as well as acting as a counterpose. The Plough promotes flexibility in the spine and hips while the Fish expands the chest and opens the throat.

PLOUGH

26

The Plough usually follows the Shoulder Stand, but it can also be practiced separately.

Having bent your knees toward your face as you descend from the Shoulder Stand, carefully extend your legs over your head until your toes touch the floor.

Continue supporting your back with your hands and try to make your back and legs as straight as you can to improve your position.

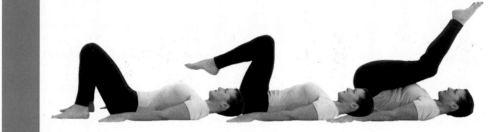

FISH

27

Lying on your back with your legs extended, take a few minutes to settle down after performing the Shoulder Stand.

Lift your torso so that you can bring your arms in a little and place your hands, palms down, under your buttocks. Your hands should not touch.

Supporting yourself on your elbows, raise your upper back off the floor, arching backward.

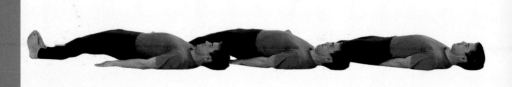

how's it going?

The Plough requires some flexibility so work in stages. You need not, for example, lower your feet to the floor when you begin; instead, straighten your knees but keep your feet off the floor until you feel able to go farther. Also, your breathing will be restricted as your chest compresses while you hold this pose. If the Fish is practiced correctly, some pressure will be placed on the neck, so it is not advised for anyone with weakness in the neck.

⌃ how's it going?

To complete the posture, straighten your arms along the floor and interlink your fingers, palms together.

Hold the position for up to 10 breaths, breathing comfortably.

To come out of the pose, replace your hands on your back and return to a supine position in the same way as in the Shoulder Stand (see pp. 70–71).

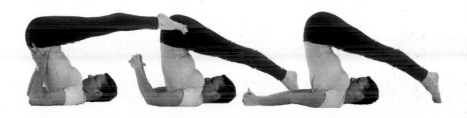

Tilt your head back until the top of your head rests on the floor. Stop if you feel any discomfort in your neck.

Finally, bring your hands to your chest, palms together, and fingers pointing upward. Breathe slowly and deeply and hold for several breaths.

To come out, place your elbows back on the floor to support your upper body. Lift your head up and gently lower yourself. Relax for a few moments with your hands by your sides.

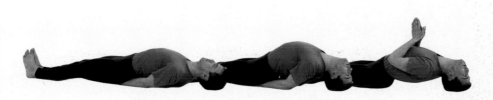

▶▶

28-29

the asanas continued

The Canoe stretches and strengthens the arms, shoulders, back, and the backs of the legs, while the Cobra improves spinal flexibility and opens up the chest.

CANOE

28

Lie down on your stomach with your arms extended in front of you, your hands shoulder-width apart, and your forehead touching the mat.

As you inhale, lift your right arm and left leg, stretching your hand forward and your foot backward.

Check that your elbows, wrists, and knees remain straight and that you do not stretch your arm out to the side. Also keep your fingers pointing directly out in front of you.

COBRA

29

Lie on your stomach, with your arms by your sides, your feet slightly apart and your forehead touching the mat.

Bend your elbows and place your hands under your shoulders, fingers forward and elbows tucked in by your sides. It is important that your elbows remain by your sides and do not stick outward.

Inhale as you lift your head and your upper body, taking your weight on your hands. Make sure that your abdomen remains in contact with the floor.

how's it going?

Bending your back also means stretching and opening the front of your body, evident in the Cobra. Check that your abdomen remains on the floor so that, in order to lift up, you have to bend your back. Do not be tempted to force yourself up by pushing hard on your hands; instead, learn to relax your back so that it curves comfortably, to imitate a striking Cobra.

⌃ how's it going?

Exhale as you lower your arm and leg, then repeat with your left arm and right leg.

Then raise your right arm and right leg, followed by your left arm and left leg.

Finally, raise both arms, both legs, and your head, resting on your stomach. Then come down gently.

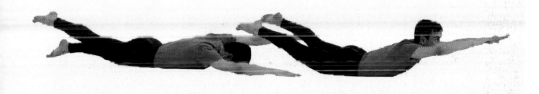

Allow your back to relax and bend as you come up. Visualize extending your breastbone forward. You may either straighten your arms or keep your elbows bent.

Hold the pose, breathing slowly, allowing your back to curve farther if this feels comfortable. Take care not to hunch your shoulders—keep them well down.

Come out of the posture slowly on an exhalation.

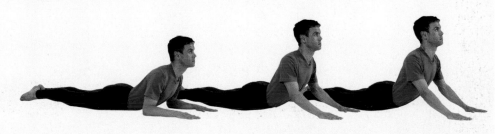

▶▶

30-31

the asanas continued

The Locust strengthens the back and the legs. The Bow, in addition to promoting flexibility in the spine, also works strongly on the arms and shoulders.

LOCUST

30 Lie on your stomach with your chin on the mat and your arms by your sides.

Make fists with your hands and place them under your hips, thumbs inward.

In this pose, the active movement is carried out on an exhalation and not an inhalation.

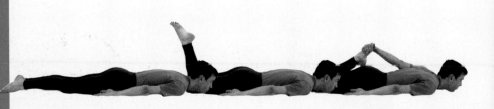

BOW

31 Lie on your stomach with your chin on the mat and your arms by your sides.

Note that in this posture, as in the Locust, you move as you exhale.

Inhale as you bend your knees and take hold of your feet or ankles with your hands.

how's it going?

While practicing the Locust, try to prevent your pelvis from twisting by maintaining the contact between your pelvis, your hands, and the floor. This is important while lifting your leg. If you have knee problems, practice the Bow with care; in this flexed position, the knees become more vulnerable as the leg muscles are used strongly to lift the body into the back bend.

⏶ how's it going?

Exhale as you raise and stretch your left leg, keeping your knee straight and lifting from the hip.

Lower your leg as you inhale, and repeat the movement three times before doing the same with your right leg. Then turn your toes under and gently push your body forward a little.

As you exhale, strongly swing both legs upward, checking that your knees remain straight. Hold briefly and lower them as you inhale. Release your hands and finish by resting for a few moments with your forehead against the floor.

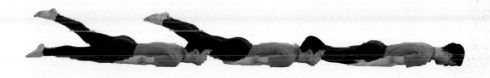

Exhale as you press your feet backward as if you were trying to straighten your knees. This will have the effect of raising your upper body and thighs off the floor so that you are resting on your stomach.

Keep your head up and try to lift your upper body and thighs as high as you can. Release as you inhale and repeat twice more.

When you become more familiar with the Bow, improve the posture by keeping your knees and ankles as close together as you can.

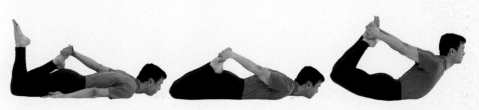

▶▶

32-33

the asanas continued

Alternate Nostril Breathing is not strictly an asana, but can usefully be included at the end of your session to balance and quieten the body in preparation for Savasana (Corpse pose), the period of relaxation at the end of your practice.

ALTERNATE NOSTRIL BREATHING

32

Choose a comfortable sitting position, either in a chair or on the floor. Close your eyes and place your right hand against your face. Place your index and middle fingers against your forehead, either straight or bent. Your head should be upright; do not let it drop forward.

Press your thumb gently against your right nostril to close it and inhale slowly and deeply through the left nostril. Press your ring finger against the left nostril so that both nostrils are closed, and briefly hold your breath. Release your thumb and exhale through the right nostril only.

Without moving your fingers, inhale through the right nostril, pause with both nostrils closed, release the left nostril, and exhale. This completes one round. Continue this method of breathing practice for several rounds. Complete the practice by removing your hand and breathing through both nostrils in a normal rhythm for 10 breaths.

how's it going?

Alternate Nostril Breathing is one of a series of techniques called *pranayama* for controlling the energy of the body by the control of the breath. If you have high blood pressure, do not hold your breath as suggested, but follow the inhalation directly with an exhalation. In Savasana, your body is placed in an open, neutral position in which it can relax completely. Because your body weight is supported by the floor, you enable tight muscles and stiff joints to soften, your blood to circulate freely, and your nervous system to function as fully as possible.

⬆ how's it going?

SAVASANA

33

Lie on your back, your body straight, your arms by your sides, and your knees bent. Start to straighten your legs one at a time until your feet are hip-width apart. If you have a back problem, keep your knees bent so your lower back stays in contact with the floor.

Lengthen the back of your neck so that your chin is tucked in rather than sticking upward. Some people may find it more comfortable to support their head on a small cushion. Place your arms away from your sides, palms facing upward.

Check your body for any areas of stress or tension. Your arms and legs should feel heavy, your shoulders and back relaxed, and your face soft. Don't forget to relax your jaw as well.

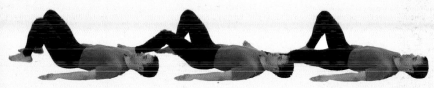

Close your eyes and focus on the peaceful, rhythmic flow of your breathing. You should feel your stomach gently rising and falling as you inhale and exhale.

Extend each exhalation so that it becomes a little longer than the inhalation and imagine your whole body letting go of tightness and tension as you exhale. Enjoy the short pause following the exhalation, when your whole body is still, before you breathe in again.

When it is time to end your period of relaxation, come out of it slowly by waking up different parts of your body in turn and finishing by opening your eyes and rolling over onto your right side before you sit up.

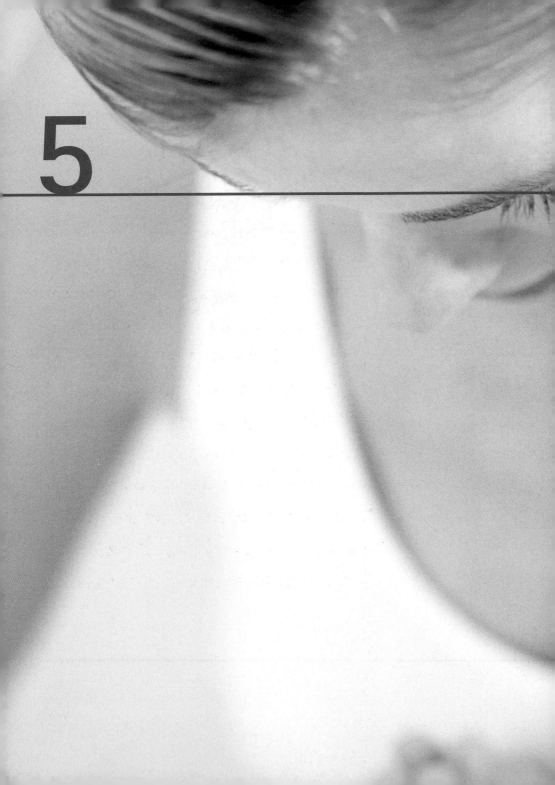

5

meditation

Meditation is essential to yoga and should be an integral part of your regular practice. Effective meditation builds slowly from simple techniques and has a clear goal: finding the stillness of your inner nature. This is achieved through a combination of correct posture, conscious, peaceful breathing, relaxation, visualization and concentration, and the power of repetition, or mantras. More importantly, the key to meditation is realizing that it is not a matter of doing it in a right or wrong way, but finding your own way to enjoy the blissful state that it brings.

stilling the mind

We have seen that the whole essence of yoga is the stilling of the mind. All the different types of yoga ultimately lead to this end. Classical (or Raja) yoga outlines the specific steps you need to take to reach this goal. Many people want to ignore this aspect of yoga, thinking that the asanas are sufficient to lead to health and well-being. The truth is that health and well-being depend upon a highly flexible mind, capable of single-mindedness and having the ability to let go.

In order to work toward this disciplined mind, all our activities, from the simplest to the most complicated, need to be coordinated. So while the capacity to meditate effectively has to be acquired gradually, learning simple meditative techniques is important from the very start.

Many of our difficulties in life stem from an inability to concentrate. Yoga meditation techniques can help us to improve focus our minds.

meditation and concentration

We all need the ability to concentrate, and are encouraged to develop this skill from an early age, yet no one provides us with any training on how to achieve it. Our chattering minds produce and process all sorts of information, but bringing it all under our own direction is difficult.

The asana is an easy object lesson in purposeful concentration, because our mental processes are directed to a physical movement and linked to a helpful image. For example, a sitting forward stretch, in which you seek to clasp your feet with legs extended, can often be much easier if you visualize someone you love in front of you. Each of you is holding out your hands to the other but you do not quite touch. Each time you breathe out—the relaxing aspect of breathing—you feel your hands moving forward to touch those of your loved one. This quite simple visualization can make a tremendous difference to your physical performance without the danger of overstraining.

meditation and relaxation

Meditation follows naturally from relaxation. The asana used for relaxation is *Savasana*, or the pose of the corpse (see p. 79). This prone position allows you to let go mentally while at the same time enjoying the utmost physical relaxation. Why, then, do we not use this position for

meditation? The answer is that while relaxation and meditation are closely related, they are not the same.

Meditation requires a wholly balanced physical tension and this can best be achieved with the trunk in an upright position. The breathing, too, is slightly different. In relaxation, the abdominal muscles are free to allow gentle movement of the stomach; in meditation, these muscles are held gently but firmly so that you breathe with your diaphragm (see "Conscious breathing," p.84).

PRACTICING VISUALIZATION AND CONCENTRATION

1 Choose a subject for your visualization in advance.

2 Sit on the floor or erect in a chair, your feet flat on the floor, and your head balanced. Shake any tension out of your muscles and join your hands in your lap.

3 Breathe steadily through your nose (with your mouth closed) for a few minutes, concentrating on your breathing.

4 Allow the subject of your visualization, as well as the feelings you associate with it, to form in your mind. Hold the image for a few minutes, while maintaining your steady breathing.

5 Then open your eyes and try to retain the feeling that the visualization brought.

6 Practice this several times a week; you will find that the amount of time you can concentrate on the image will quickly increase.

conscious breathing

Peaceful awareness of breathing is essential. The Buddhists have developed this to a fine art in a process they call "conscious breathing," which uses the diaphragm while meditating. This means that you gently control your trunk muscles so that your chest does not heave and your abdomen does not move up and down.

Your diaphragm—the toughest layer of striated muscle in your body—is situated at the bottom of your ribs, attached to the lowest one. This is where you should feel movement in meditation: right in the middle of your trunk. As you breathe with your diaphragm, it acts like an engine to keep energy flowing throughout your body and brain.

breathing techniques

Sit correctly (see below) and comfortably with your eyes gently closed. Some people advocate meditating with the eyes open but, generally, closing your eyes is preferable. Become aware of your breath, saying "rising" to yourself as you breathe in, and "falling" as you breathe out, all the time observing sound, movement, and position. Another popular method is to count slowly from one to 10 as you breathe in, then back down to one as you breathe out.

As for timing, meditation can last from a few minutes to—in extreme instances—hours. About five minutes is good for a beginner, but resist any temptation to look at your watch, other than before or after. Letting your mind wander onto how long you have been meditating is not helpful. Gradually, you can increase the length of time you sit, but don't rush it. Most people who regularly meditate at home will take between 15 and 30 minutes.

POSITION AND BREATHING

It does not matter whether you meditate sitting on the floor or upright on a chair. Sitting in a cross-legged position, or back on your toes on the floor, are especially suitable, however, as they restrict blood flow in the legs and feet, thus stimulating it in the upper parts of the body.

The position of your hands plays a part. Place them in your lap with one cupped in the palm of the other, or place them on your knees, with the tip of each thumb placed against the tip of each index finger.

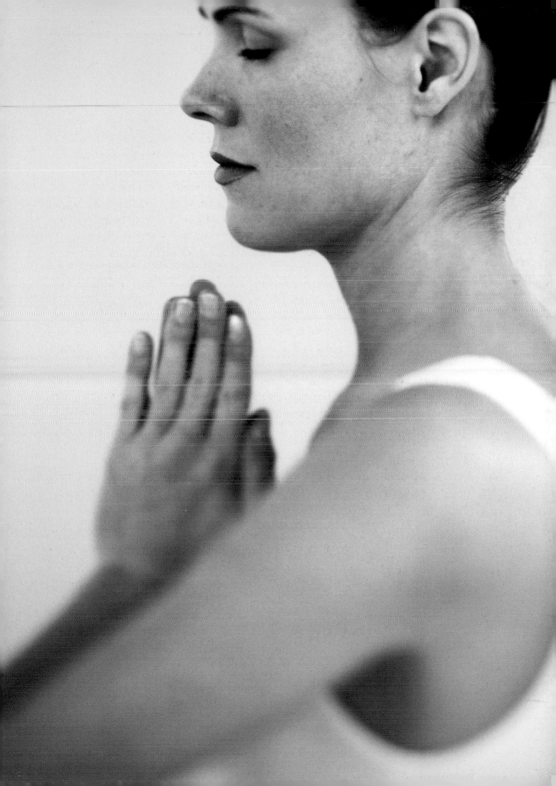

letting go

As you try to focus on your awareness of your breathing, other thoughts will intrude, but try simply to let them come and go without emotion, maintaining the rising and falling breathing pattern throughout. Often, if ignored, these thoughts will float away again. If not, examine them quietly and then dismiss them. Gradually, the unneeded thoughts will lessen and the calmness, rhythm, and peace of breathing will take over.

The goal of meditation is to release your mind from your everyday thoughts and to know the stillness of your inner nature. With continued patience and practice, you will begin to experience this wonderful state of being.

meditation techniques

There are countless meditation techniques, but all the classical ones begin with some process to establish awareness of the rhythm and peace of the breathing. One of the best-known techniques is mantra (see "The power of repetition," p. 87), but there are many other ways to calm the mind. The late Swami Sivananda urged disciples to use the same visualization process as described above, but using their most revered figure—Christ, the Buddha, Krishna, or a living person with whom you especially identify, as the subject. This should not just be like looking at a statue; there needs to be a feeling of empathy—a two-way process—between meditator and subject.

Ultimately, there is no "right" or "wrong" way of meditating. While we are all part of a universal whole, we are also individuals with different outlooks and tastes. Study with an open mind and follow the procedure with which you feel most comfortable, providing it fits in with the basics: comfortable upright trunk; hands linked or in a classical linking of thumb and index finger, awareness of the quiet, rhythmical breath at all times. Once you have fulfilled these basics—let go.

People with stressful lifestyles are increasingly utilizing the powerful visualization techniques of yoga to gain a more balanced perspective and introduce a sense of peace into their lives.

THE POWER OF REPETITION

1 Mantra—the repetition of a word or phrase during meditation—is a powerful technique for stilling the mind. It is claimed that certain words, such as *om*, have a special value, but it is not so much the words used as the spirit in which they are recited.

2 You can use an obvious and simple word, such as "peace." However, this is such a common word that you may find it slipping away. If instead you say *ahimsa* (the absence of violence), the very strangeness of the term is likely to keep it in the forefront of your mind.

3 Whatever phrase you choose to repeat, it should be carried through with constant attention to your breathing, so that it becomes rhythmical, in unison with the rising and falling process.

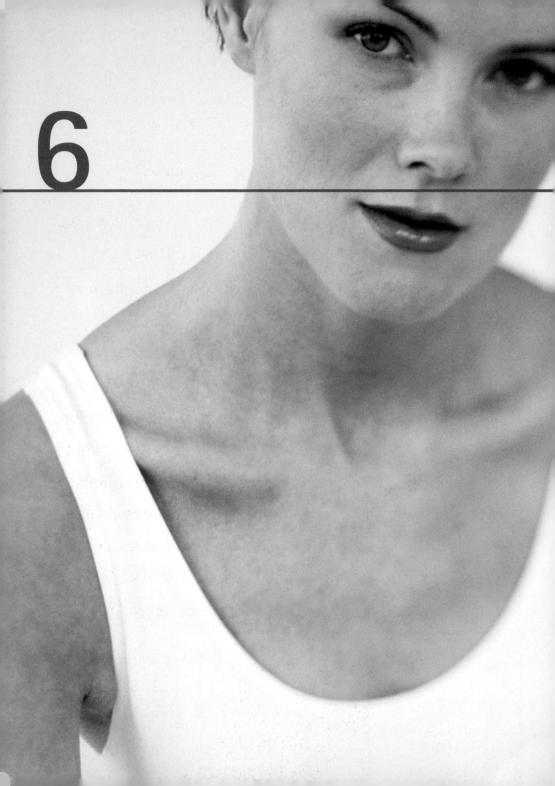

6

yoga in everyday life

As we have seen, the greatest benefits of yoga are to be enjoyed by adopting a holistic approach that encompasses regular physical practice, concentration, contemplation, meditation, and ethical living. In this final section, we examine briefly how, through perseverance and accepting responsibility for our own lives, yoga can lead to the ultimate goal of attaining enlightenment through stillness. As demonstrated by the practitioners of the different schools of yoga throughout the ages, this can be a lifetime's work. But work in this context, of course, means true, profound joy.

holistic benefits

As we have seen, yoga is fundamentally holistic and works on the premise that mind and body are parts of an integrated whole. Yoga also applies to all aspects of our lives, not just to yoga classes or practicing asanas. The great thing about the mental and physical union of yoga is that we feel the benefits of the discipline—and it is a discipline—from the beginning, provided this holistic approach is taken.

looking at illness

In the West we are increasingly used to being offered instant solutions to our problems, but that is not the way our bodies, or our lives in general, work. For example, those using yoga as an antidote to a particular health problem may find that they make quick progress in solving the problem, then find that this motivates them further. The approach of the Hatha yoga session helps those starting out along the path to feel refreshed and better, both mentally and physically, but it is important to realize that we need perseverance if we are really to benefit from yoga and successfully adopt its principles and practice into our lives.

So the benefits of yoga are often felt very quickly and can stay with us for the rest of our lives. However, it is wise to be aware of the possibility that your progress may slow at times. If this is the case, remember that any problems you are on the right path to solving often develop over a long period of time and while their modification or even removal can take place, it can never be an overnight affair. So maintain a gentle, methodical approach.

We need to keep in mind just why we are practicing yoga and to make sure we always realize its all-inclusive approach. Just why we fall ill or have physical problems is a highly complex matter and no one has all the answers. Genes, heredity, and environmental factors all have a role, but it is clear that while we need to know what is going wrong, physically and mentally, the important thing is to examine why and how we are facing up to it. We have a great deal of responsibility for ourselves in most instances. In fact, yogis believe that we have total responsibility for our personal situations. Practicing yoga enables us to clear our minds, pinpoint our objectives, and direct our lives.

So it is important that we establish self-responsibility. Books and teachers can offer detailed programs to follow, but the best way of moving forward is to study the principles of yoga and then relate them to our own particular situations, rather than just following a prescribed path. The art of yogic living is based upon finding the correct balance between expressing our individuality and understanding our place in the universe.

Yoga must be a step-by-step process. Even the great yogis realize this

PERSONALITY AWARENESS

The sages believed that three threads, or *gunas*, interlink with the physical and spiritual to produce life. Pure, good, life force, known as *sattva*, is the first thread. The second thread is *rajas*—energy or mobility. The third thread is the force of inertia or darkness, called *tamas*. All three forces exist in every aspect of life.

The *gunas* can be used as a model to explain how we react to situations and what our personalities are like. Through this understanding, we can recognize and modify how we behave by bringing the three *gunas* into balance.

Personalities with an excess of *rajasic* force tend to be competitive, stressed, and likely to react to problems in an irritable way. They may suffer from stress related health problems.

Personalities with too much *tamasic* force often feel powerless and unable to remedy a situation when something goes wrong. They may suffer from depression and lack of energy.

Personalities that exhibit *sattva* are the ones who can strike a balance between the two. Yoga practice increases our tendency to behave in a *sattvic* way—dispassionately and balanced. This can be a lifetime's work.

in their own lives as well as in their teachings. An eminent Indian yogi, who had suffered ill-health, was asked how he was now. His reply was that "I am as well as I let myself be." It is this realization of the role we play in our own lives that is important to understand.

ethics
The ethical basis of yoga—the *yamas* and *niyamas* (see pp. 20–21)—provides the framework for adopting yoga into everyday life. Their message—that we should lead a peaceful life of respect for ourselves and others—is part of the oneness of yoga. The result of our behaving in the way they suggest will benefit our own lives physically and mentally, as well as the lives of others.

This is not as easy as it sounds. The desire to avenge a wrong that has been done to us, an urge to take more than we are entitled to, and so on, can be tempting. It manifests itself in what Professor Hans Selye described as "distress"—stress that is harmful, as distinct from that which is helpful in motivating us. The thoughtful practice of the asanas, linked with gradually learning to meditate, provides the basis for harmony in which cooperation and self-fulfilment take the place of actions that are harmful to ourselves and others.

So yoga is not just a leisure activity but the process of losing tension, feeling released and at one with the world and those in it—a priceless goal.

the ultimate goal

Over the many years during which the approach to life we call yoga developed, the sages realized that although ultimately all is one, individuals have varied ways of reaching a common goal—an idea often called "unity in diversity." So other types of yoga developed as an adjunct to the Hatha yoga and Raja yoga we have seen in this book.

other approaches

We have already looked at Patanjali's Raja yoga (see pp. 18-19). This is the approach linking all the aspects of yoga, which we termed Classical yoga. However, it is not the only approach. Some people naturally have a devout nature and they are called "Bhakti yogis" (after the Sanskrit term for devotion). A third approach is "Karma yoga." The word karma is the Sanskrit for fate or destiny, and it is used here to describe outcomes arising from our actions.

BEING STILL

Stillness is at the core of the yogic process. Developing stillness of mind, emotions, and body takes time. The story is told of a student who approached a swami and said, "I want to devote myself wholly to yoga. How long will it take me to reach a truly advanced stage?" The swami replied, "About five years." The student exclaimed, "But I will work hard every day. How long, master?" The swami replied, "About 10 years." Now the student jumped up and down. "You don't understand," he said, "I'll work harder and harder. How long?" With a smile the swami replied, "About 20 years."

It is thus similar to the law of cause and effect.

The yamas and niyamas come into play again with Karma yoga. Karma yoga shows us that how we live day by day (that is, following the yamas and niyamas) will determine the way our lives unfold. This book offers a starting point to yoga using Hatha yoga, but not all the styles of yoga use the asanas. For example, Mahatma Gandhi was a yogi but he did not include Hatha yoga asanas in his practice; however, for the great majority of us, Hatha yoga offers a tangible and rewarding approach to yoga.

At this point it is important to remember that yoga is not a religion. There are links and parallels with the teachings of all the main religions of the world, including Hinduism, Buddhism, Sikhism, Jainism, Judaism, and Christianity. Yoga conceives all religious beliefs as essentially one in spirit and promotes this understanding in all its practices. As we have already seen, yoga came about through the sages' realization that the finest way to gain knowledge is to be still. The knowledge arising from stillness is the whole basis of yoga.

the right emphasis

In fact, the subject of yoga is the subject of life itself, so the words beginner, intermediate, or advanced have very little meaning, since there is

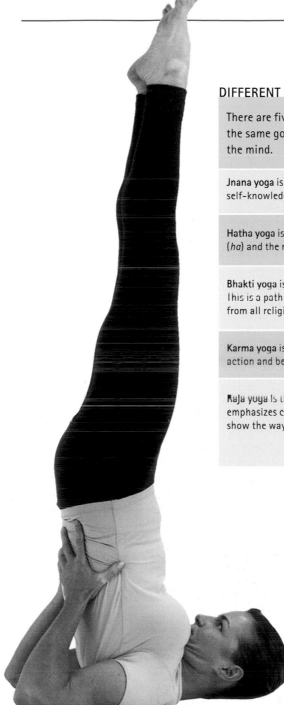

DIFFERENT SCHOOLS OF YOGA

There are five main styles of yoga, all of which share the same goal—enlightenment through the stilling of the mind.

Jnana yoga is the path of sacred wisdom, and emphasizes self-knowledge through religious and philosophical inquiry.

Hatha yoga is the yoga of balanced force. It balances the sun (*ha*) and the moon (*tha*).

Bhakti yoga is the path of worship and spiritual devotion. This is a path naturally followed by saints and mystics from all religions.

Karma yoga is the path of action. It emphasizes selfless action and behavior.

Raja yoga is the "King of yogas" (see pp. 18–19) and emphasizes controlling the mind. The eight limbs of yoga show the way to achieving this aim.

no real end-point to be reached. The essential thing is to realize what is going on in our minds and lives. It is hard to say that we shouldn't feel satisfaction when we find our performance of the asanas improving, but the real improvement lies in the totality of the performance. Mental calmness is far more important than physical dexterity—although the two can go hand in hand. Physical suppleness naturally has its value, but the real test comes when we start to see changes in how we deal with the everyday challenges of life.

making progress

For most of us progress will involve finding a teacher with whom we have empathy. While good training is important, the teacher must be able to share and communicate the unity that is yoga. Excellent performance of the asanas will always take second place.

In this book we have touched on different aspects of yoga. We must at all times remember that the ultimate unity does not mean that we do not have individual differences of approach. Therefore, in developing our yoga, we must beware of placing too much emphasis on learning all the correct Sanskrit terms and theories, as if being tested in an examination. Even those studying to become teachers need to have a good introductory period before beginning to learn the subject in earnest. The adjudicators of any reputable training program will note the difference between a student taking a simple but sincere approach and one who is sprinkling his or her papers with Sanskrit terms and complex concepts.

So yoga is firmly based on the sense of wonder, the sense of peace that comes when body, mind, and spirit come together, in the asanas (poses), in *pranayama* (controlled breathing), in *darana* (concentration), and in *dyana* (meditation).

As this union is developed, so it moves on from the specific periods of practice to the whole of the day. This linkage of the different aspects of our existence becomes a central part of our life. People often feel that their lives change for the better when they begin practicing yoga.

We need to realize this essential unity and live our lives accordingly. Those tempted to dismiss such a concept as untrue, should realize that many scientists and clinicians, such as Albert Einstein and Bernie Siegel, discussed at the beginning of the book, have had corresponding ideas.

Yoga offers us the opportunity to experience life in a new and healthy manner. As it is practiced, the yogic lifestyle becomes more useful to the situations we face in our lives. As we master one challenge, we move to the next. The expression "be here now" reminds us that our concepts of the past and future are integrally related to our current attitudes. If we are living fully in the moment, we have no need to be overly concerned about the future. We follow our inner promptings to enlightenment.

The joy of yoga is experienced as we desire to learn more and to share the many benefits that we have gained. In the West alone, the number of people practicing yoga is now many millions, many led by non-Indian teachers who recognize the value of yogic practices. Even in India, the home of yoga, there has been a great revival of interest in the subject.

glossary

Ahimsa:
The absence of violence in thought, word, or deed. It is one of the five *yamas*. See also *niyamas*.

Asana:
The postures of yoga. In the eight limbs of yoga, the asanas are the third limb.

Ashtanga yoga:
The eight limbs of yoga in the Classical yoga system described by Patanjali.

Bhakti yoga:
One of the schools of yoga that emphasizes the path of worship and spiritual devotion. It is naturally followed by holy men.

Brahman:
The ultimate universal force or the ultimate spirit of the universe.

Darana:
The development of single-minded concentration, the first step in meditation and the sixth limb of the eight limbs of Classical yoga.

Dyana:
The process of contemplation and meditation, which is at the heart of yoga. It is the seventh limb of the eight limbs of Classical yoga.

Gunas:
The three threads, or qualities, that, intertwined with *prakriti* and *purusha*, produce all life.

Hatha yoga:
The yoga of balanced force. It includes the asanas along with the mental aspects of yoga.

Jnana yoga:
One of the schools of yoga that emphasizes the path of wisdom through intellectual inquiry.

Karma yoga:
One of the schools of yoga that emphasizes the path of action. This action should be made up of selfless behavior.

Mantra:
A sacred thought or prayer repeated during meditation and used as a technique for stilling the mind.

Niyamas:
The ethical rules, or "five actions," that guide our conduct toward others. They are the second of the eight limbs of Classical yoga and complement the *yamas*.

Prakriti:
The sum total of material matter in the universe.

Prana:
The ultimate life force, linked with the breath.

Pranayama:
Controlling the breath to stimulate the life force. See *prana*.

Pratyahara:
The necessity of not being a slave to the senses of the outer world, and the need to examine the essential inner world contained within us all. It is the fifth of the eight limbs of Classical yoga.

Purusha:
The force of universal consciousness. The sages saw that *purusha* was interwoven with *prakriti*, the material matter of the universe.

Raja yoga:
The "King of yogas," otherwise called Classical yoga. It places emphasis on controlling the mind.

Rajas:
The force of energy or mobility. Also the second thread of the *gunas*.

Samadi:
The ultimate state of deep meditation. It is the last of the eight limbs of Classical yoga.

Santosha:
The power of equanimity or dispassion.

Sattva:
Pure, illuminating, positive life force. Also the first thread of the *gunas*.

Tamas:
The force of inertia or darkness. Also the third thread of the *gunas*.

Yamas:
The five ethical rules governing our own actions and the first of the eight limbs of Classical yoga.

index

acknowledgments
Many thanks to Sweatshop U.K. for kindly providing clothing.